Paramedic Buff To Burnt

To order additional copies, please contact us.
BookSurge, LLC
www.booksurge.com
1-866-308-6235
orders@booksurge.com

Paramedic
Buff To Burnt

By New York City Paramedic
George Steffensen

Cover Picture by Tom Hobbs
Graphic Design by Anthony D. Matthews

2005

Paramedic Buff To Burnt

Editing by
Jennifer Lape
DM of the missing:

To my wife Luci, who has saved me, and has been there for me through the good times and bad. To the kids Jennifer, Richie, Rachael, and Hollie, thank you for your love and support. To my Grandson Dustin, thank you for your love and support too. Thanks to those who have been there for me, on the jobs and with this book.

In loving memory of
my Mother,
Norah Steffensen
and
my Aunt,
Margaret Johnston.

BY NEW YORK CITY PARAMEDIC

George Steffensen

Paramedic buff to burnt is a book about paramedics told by a highly decorated New York City paramedic with over fifteen years on the streets. It will start with my training and then take you from being a rookie paramedic to being an old-timer (or dinosaur as we call it). I will share some of my thoughts about the training, the different people I have dealt with over the many years and the changes I have gone through from when I first became a paramedic until now, seventeen years later. Most importantly, it will cover some of the interesting and crazy calls I have responded to over these long years. At times it will be a bit unbelievable! As we all know, truth is stranger than fiction.

The term buff refers to a new paramedic, excited about his or her job, excited about saving lives, doing good, helping people. Using all the new skills acquired in paramedic school. Starting intravenous lines, pushing drugs, intubations, electrocardiograms and shocking people with your defibrillator.

Then (if you are lucky) saving someone. Yes, we will be saving people. Unfortunately, we will be losing people too. The best you can do is to do your job well and the outcome is up to God or Whomever you believe in.

Burnt, on the other hand, is the paramedic who has been on the streets too long. He is the medic who doesn't care about the patients any longer. The only good job for this medic is the cancellation or the unfounded. He no longer gets excited about the trauma jobs. Not interested if he just saved a life, no more adrenalin pumping, every call is just a bother. He just does it as he is now stuck in this "hell hole of a job," too old and too tired to go onto something else.

Fortunately for me, I may be a little toasted but far from burnt. I guess I am a lucky one. I have been a medic over 17 years, 15 of them here in New

York City. I still love my job…despite the times you catch me complaining. Most EMTs (Emergency Medical Technicians) and paramedics go through their whole careers being great EMTs and medics without any recognition for their life saving work. I on the other hand have had more then my share of recognition.

At times we have all been in some very dangerous situations. Putting our lives in jeopardy to help some stranger. People recognize firemen and police as heroes, as I do too. I also recognize the men and women of the Emergency Medical Services as heroes too. I know the dangers that we have faced and the dangers we will continue to face.

To my fellow emergency medical technicians and paramedics…thank you for a job well done! So let me take you on this trip through the life of a paramedic. Let me bring you into the action…the highs of saving a life to the lows of losing a loved one.

BY NEW YORK CITY PARAMEDIC GEORGE STEFFENSEN

MY STORY

I started as a paramedic in 1987. My first job was with a small private service doing mostly non-emergency transports. This was not very exciting. It wasn't easy starting out as a new medic. Most places want some experience. I applied to a fly car service in Rockland County, based out of a hospital. This would turn out to be the break I needed. They were starting to expand and needed help. Although they would have preferred a medic with experience they took a chance with me. They always put me with experienced medics, and the ones they put me with were great. No one likes the new guys that much and being put with a new medic (believe me) can be very trying.

I look back to those medics who took me under their wings and helped me. To this day I can't thank them enough for what they taught me and the way they redirected my actions, with respect. Not to make me feel like an idiot or embarrass me. I don't want to name them, as I'm afraid I might forget a name and that would not be right. Let me say to the medics out there who have helped me back in my rookie days: THANK YOU. To the medics that were too cool to remember what being new was and treated me like an idiot, well I have two words for you too. I'll just say those two words are not happy birthday.

During the early days of being a medic, I was the buff. I couldn't wait to get the calls. I was eager to save someone, to help and use these new skills.

The problem was that I was new and these so called skills were far from skillful. Starting IVs always looked easy for the old timers but for me it was hit and miss, more misses then hits to be honest. Responding to calls was great; preparing in my mind what I might be doing by the type of call the dispatcher gave us. I would watch my partners and try to see their way of getting the history from the patient. This skill is not as fancy as doing the IVs or any of the other cool things you see medics do on TV but all the IVs and all the medications we carry are useless if you don't know what you are treating. It takes great skill to differentiate between pulmonary edema and pneumonia. It will also take me some time to know that just because I have drugs and all this fancy equipment that every patient won't need a complete work up.

This is a far cry from the burnt medic that feels no one is sick enough to use any equipment on them. As a new medic I carried all kinds of stuff. I had the big buff belt that was somewhat like Batman's. You will always know the newer medic from the old timer by the amount of stuff they have on their buff belt. The old-timer or burnt medic for sure won't even have a buff belt. The only belt he will be wearing is the one that holds his pants up.

I don't wear a buff belt anymore but I do carry an oxygen wrench, and trauma shears. They are tied together by a hospital wristband and then the O2 key tucks into my waistband. One of my partners had it like that and I liked the fact that I had these things close at hand. There are times when your oxygen tank starts to leak or you need your shears quickly so I still keep them on me. Other than that everything else I will need is with the rest of the equipment. And the stethoscope not being around the neck really feels much better.

The other changes that come will come over time. The way you feel after a call where you have lost someone. The thoughts you have after you have seen something really gruesome. The amount of adrenalin rush you get during an exciting job. The lack of adrenalin rush after you have been on the streets too long. The way you care about the patients to the way you start to care more about yourself.

In the beginning the patient comes first, but with time that starts to change. After awhile all the abuse get starts to get you frustrated.

If you think that being a medic is going to be saving people and using your skills to do good, you will be greatly disappointed. From my experience, medics and EMTs don't get burnt out by the exciting jobs or the horrors that they deal with, but more from the abuse of the system. The calls for the unconscious who will be the drunk on the sidewalk. The cardiac that will be the kid with a cold but will come in as a cardiac because this kid had a history of a heart murmur when he was born.

You will risk your life fighting traffic to arrive to someone walking around in their apartment telling you they just don't feel well. Their doctor told them to meet him at the hospital. The other thing, after almost killing yourselves getting to the call, there will always be someone to complain: "What took you so long?" There is so much more abuse of the system but I really think you get the point. What is truly the case is that no one really cares anyway. They think of themselves and don't care about the possible consequences of using an ambulance when not necessary to save the three dollars on cab fare.

If you can put all this behind you and know that ninety percent of your work will be a fancy cab ride you will be all right.

With that said, the remaining ten percent does matter. Sometimes you don't have to do much, just your being there to these people or their family members will mean a lot. There have been times in my life that I have run into someone, or a family member of someone that I have helped. Their words of thanks really touched me and have made me proud of my work. One time I was at my daughter's school for Meet-The-Teachers night. As we were leaving a woman came over to me and my daughter. She said that I had saved her husband when he was having a heart attack. She just wanted to thank me. It really made me feel great and proud, especially because my young daughter was there. I don't think that I did anything that important to save him, but I did take him to the hospital. This is what I was saying, how we touch people just from our being there. It made her feel that we had helped.

Time has taught me that small things really can make a big impact on someone. I now feel almost as good after I have placed a warm blanket on someone who is cold and laying in the emergency room when they thank me as I do when they thank me after a "real job" where what I did made a difference. Making people more comfortable, especially in a time of need or when they are alone and have no one to care, that's when my caring can mean a lot. Yes, it is not heroic, but the heroic thing is just in our minds. You can get your 15 minutes of fame but when it is all done no one really cares. Just like the heroes of wars, after awhile no one remembers them. Their medals get dusty and their stories get old.

After working for a while over in Rockland and with the private service in Northern Westchester my skills as a paramedic were getting better. I went to the city to work. I applied at a hospital on the lower east side. The boss who interviewed me was an ex-Marine. This, along with my good references helped me get the spot.

Working in the city was very different for me. These guys and gals were pretty tough. They let me know right away that they were the ones in charge, and that I was the new guy. The way they approached things was a lot different then what I was used too. In time I will understand the toughness, but at the beginning it made me a bit uncomfortable.

I happen to be a big guy, which helps when you have to deal with drunks or drugged-out people who won't hesitate to take a swing at you. The amount of calls and the type of calls were very exciting to me. Being a paramedic in New York City, this is the big leagues. When I started in the city I was still pretty much a rookie, only with some experience. I started working in the city in 1989, so I had been a paramedic for almost two years. As time passes the amount of stuff on my buff belt will diminish. The rookie me would start out my shift checking to make sure every little item was there. All medications were present and they were not expired.

As time goes on the checking got to be more of a quick check. I would look at a few key items then be ready to go. Now I get in the bus look to see if there is stuff on the stretcher from the previous crew. If there is stuff on there I'm good. Ready to get my coffee before I give my first signal, which puts me available for jobs. My thinking now is that the rookie medics from the shift before already checked things. I know it must be good.

I once would think about what to do when I would get to the calls. Now I just hope that we will get cancelled or it will turn out to be unfounded. Which means no one is there on the arrival of the ambulance. The buff me couldn't wait to perform some fancy procedure. The toasty me now hopes that all I'll need to do is a quick set of vitals, and off to the hospital.

I have to admit I really do like helping people, but my enthusiasm is just a lot less. The fact that ninety percent is nonsense will take a toll on anyone. Don't laugh, you old burnt medics, I'm not that burnt. I still feel good when I have a chance to do something worthwhile. Even this past week and it has been awhile since I've done a "real job." I had some real calls and made a difference. Those are the days that remind me why I do it.

All kidding aside, being a paramedic for me has been great. Even after 17 years on the streets, I still love it. The partners to the co-workers, I'll explain the difference later. All have touched me in someway. We share some great moments, and some awful moments too. Together we get through it.

Working with the police and fire departments, I have made some close bonds with them too. The different people, from the millionaires to the Bowery bums, they all are the same underneath it all. There are some really nice ones, and some really not so nice ones. Hard to believe, but as much as we complain about picking up drunks, I know a few tough medics that cried when one of our regular drunks died one cold winter night.

The rest of this book will go over some of the calls that come to mind, some of them funny and some not so funny. Please bear with me, as I am a medic not a writer. However most writers can't tell you first hand what it is like to take someone who has no pulse, basically dead, and with their skills and training get them back to life. Not too many people know what it is like to climb under a subway train to help a stranger. I will share these stories, and hopefully you will get the feeling of what being there is all about. For me it has been an amazing experience being a medic. The people I've met, and seeing things in ways most people don't get the chance to see. Being right there in the action. When others are stopped from going closer to a disaster, we are the ones making the difference between life and death. Sounds dramatic, and it is.

BY NEW YORK CITY PARAMEDIC GEORGE STEFFENSEN

TRAINING

Paramedic training was a true challenge for me. I was a poor student in high school. I never did much work and spent most of those days hanging out. My guidance councilor recommended that I quit high school. My mom didn't like that idea and made sure I finished. After high school I joined the Marine Corps. Those drill instructors sure don't have a sense of humor. What they do have is a way to get you to grow up, and become responsible. I still joke around too much, but I did learn to try my best at what ever I do. I learned electronics in the Marines, and worked in that field for ten years. The electronic business was always changing, and layoffs were always a threat. So before this would happen to me, I wanted to change to a different field. I had been an emergency medical technician, and volunteered in my small town in Westchester.

Paramedics were starting to work in our area, and the pay wasn't bad. I figured that the parts of the human body don't change from year to year like in the electronic business. I will only needed to learn this stuff once, and I'll be good to go. I enrolled at Norwalk Community College paramedic class in 1986. They had a good reputation, and it was a program that would be paid for by the government from the G.I. Bill.

Going into the Marines was a good move. Well, it was for me anyway. Don't go running down there thinking the Marines are just fun and games. I'm sure that you have heard they are tough and put you through hell.

I can't believe that after all my lack of interest in school, at thirty-two here I am in college. My classmates are young kids. I feel out of place. These books are huge, with big words, and lots of them. My first thoughts are: you won't make it past the first week. You just squeaked past high school a long time ago. Well, let's remember that the Marines did teach me to try my best, so let's do it.

Back to the big books with those big words. Here's an example: "sympathomimetics drugs are grouped according to their receptor action." That sounds right I guess. I have lots of studying to do before I'll know what that all means.

The book stuff isn't easy for me, but I'm doing well. After a few months of this book stuff, they start sending us to hospitals to start doing rotations. Rotations are where we go to different areas of the hospitals to get some hands on experience. We went with the IV team to learn how to start intravenous lines. I remember my aunt Margaret being upset to hear that I was going around sticking people with needles. She knew how clumsy I was as a kid.

Then when she heard I was going into the operating rooms to put breathing tubes into people, that really had her nervous. It all went well. They had us practice on manikins before they let us do things to real people.

My skills were far from great, as was expected being so new. However with time and practice they improve. Learning about the different drugs we were going to give was very complicated. Mistakes at this new level can kill someone. Electrocardiograms and learning how to read their strips was fun and interesting for me, less confusing than the drugs. Here I could really see the changes from a normal EKG to one that had abnormalities. Maybe this was easier for me because of my electronics background.

Paramedic training was like a big puzzle. You had all these parts of the body. Then you had to understand how the different systems affected the others. All these drugs to speed up one thing, or slow something else down. I thought that I would never be able to get it all straight. Then just like a puzzle it all started to look like something. It started to make sense. I was understanding all the big words and understanding the workings of the body.

Now I can't wait to show how smart I am. Towards the end of training they have us do ambulance rotations. This is where we go out with experienced paramedics, and work as you would in the field. Working with these experienced paramedics was a lot of fun. It was also interesting to hear the different views about the job. I must admit they had me thinking I made a mistake. Most of the paramedics complained about the job.

It took over a year of this intense training, but now the training part is finally over. I'm ready to save the world. There is nothing more dangerous then a rookie paramedic wanting to try all these procedures and drugs on you. It is a good thing they put us with experienced medics when we first get out there.

There are two things you can't get from school no matter how hard you study. One is experience and the other is common sense. These two things are just as important as all the books and all the fancy procedures.

BY NEW YORK CITY PARAMEDIC GEORGE STEFFENSEN

ROOKIE MEDIC

Well here I am a new paramedic, ready to save the world. I have the big utility belt with all kinds of equipment a new medic needs. I have a holster for my radio, a pouch to hold my gloves. I have another place for my trauma shears. Then there is a holder for my big Mag-Lite. You also need a tourniquet hanging there; it lets people know you are a medic. A few more things you need on your utility belt are your oxygen key and the window punch. (The window punch is a handy tool that helps you gain access to a person locked in a car.) Don't forget about the 14-gauge catheters you need in your shirt pocket for the trauma jobs. Finally, around your neck will be the very expensive cardiology stethoscope.

Here is a tip for you. If the paramedic that comes to help you has all these things hanging off him, he is new. For your safety you should refuse any and all treatment. You should request transportation only. You have this right; use it. I laugh now when I think back to those early days. When I was overzealous and over-equipped. Of course I'm kidding a bit, even new medics are highly trained and will be working with someone who has been around a few days. Even as a new medic I did some good.

Most of the time patients don't need that much saving, and the ride to the hospital will be enough. It will take awhile before I come to realize that most of my calls will be boring and routine.

The stress from the job will be self-induced. As we head to a call as a rookie I start to review the protocol for whatever the dispatch information is. For example, if the call is for a difficulty breathing, I will think of the different scenarios for someone having difficulty breathing. I will consider asthma, pulmonary edema, pulmonary embolus, pulmonary hypertension, cor pulmonale, chronic obstructive pulmonary disease and hyperventilation. Then I will think of other medical problems that also can cause difficulty in breathing. By the time I get on scene I am exhausted from thinking too much.

Most of the time it will turn out to be something pretty simple. Maybe mild asthma; slight wheezing with good air exchange. We will give a breathing treatment and transport to the hospital. Nothing too fancy.

Let's talk about the unconscious call which, when working the lower east side, is a very common call. Again, the rookie medic will think of all the medical problems that can make a person unconscious. I will not list all that, as it will be too much and I'm sure you know what I mean from the difficulty breathing example. It will take awhile before I get it, that on the lower east side (and most of the city) the unconscious call would refer to the drunk passed out on the street.

Not to say that this is not some kind of emergency. This call is the type that can get you into big trouble. The truth is that even drunks on the streets have heart attacks. If you don't follow your protocols, and just assume he is just passed out from drinking, you will find that he did have a heart attack. Yes, you will find this when you are called into the medical directors office to explain why you did not follow your proper protocols for the unconscious. I am very serious so don't be lazy and be sure you do the right things. It always comes down to doing the right thing, and you will save yourself a lot of trouble.

When real jobs come in I am very excited. I can't wait to perform some procedure to help someone. Starting IVs was always a cool thing for me as a rookie medic. The cooler thing was to use a big catheter like a 14-gauge one. This size is one of the biggest, it has a very large diameter. It was always impressive on the trauma job to get two 14-gauge IVs started.

Intubation is another skill that as a rookie medic I wanted to perform. This is placing the breathing tube into the trachea. This can be very tricky. The airway is always the first thing that must be addressed. Without an airway you need not worry about anything else. So intubation is truly a skill that, when needed to be performed, is going to be the difference between the patient living or dying.

The tube has two places it can go when you are trying to place it. One is the trachea, and this happens to be the right one. This will get oxygen into the lungs. The patient's color will improve to a more pink color. This also gives you access to give medications, also another important factor of intubation, especially if you do not have IV access.

The other place the tube can go is the esophagus. This is the wrong place. It is not bad to misplace the tube as long as you check the tube placement. You must recognize it when it is in the wrong place and remove it quickly. The way to check proper placement is to listen to the stomach, and then both lungs. If you don't hear it in the stomach and you hear it equally in both lungs, you did it right.

If you have misplaced it, and continue to ventilate the patient, the air will be going into the stomach. The patient's color will change to blue from lack of oxygen. At this point things will only get worse. The next thing you can count on is (due to all this pressure building in the stomach) the contents of the stomach will have to go somewhere. That somewhere will be back up the misplaced tube, and all this vomit will come shooting out like a volcano. After this happens, trying to remove and replace the tube is only short of impossible.

I hope I've made the point of how important intubation is, and the consequences of what can happen if it is not done correctly.

Defibrillating people is another exciting procedure rookie medics like to do. This one is pretty easy. The good thing about defibrillating someone is that their condition can only improve. Defibrillation is reserved for the person in cardiac arrest. Cardiac arrest means no heartbeat, basically dead, so you can't kill a corpse. This is why I said that this procedure that can only improve the patients condition.

The other procedure that medics do that emergency medical technicians can't is pushing drugs. This is fun for the new medic popping the caps off the "shooters" and pushing the drugs.

Until you have given every drug in your drug box at least once, you don't feel like an experienced medic. Don't tell anyone, but in all my years on the streets, there are still a few I haven't pushed.

Yikes. I wonder if some of those patients that didn't make it should have gotten the drugs I haven't pushed yet. Do you think the oxytocin would have made the difference? Nahh, just kidding.

As a rookie medic, I will get the chance to do all this and more. My partners will help me get a better understanding of what is going on. Right now, I'm the tail wagging the dog. Excited and naive about this new work of being a paramedic.

BY NEW YORK CITY PARAMEDIC GEORGE STEFFENSEN

SHOOTINGS

MY FIRST SHOOTING

Shootings are interesting calls with lots of action. Working in the city gave me the opportunity to respond to a number of these calls. Looking back to my first shooting when I was a buff, it has still stayed pretty fresh in my mind.

It was sometime in the afternoon when my partner and I were dispatched to the shooting. I know I've said this in the other chapters, but as a new medic I would always go through what I might have to do per protocol. I would remind myself of important things to remember from training. With a gunshot you need to not only treat the first wound you see, but also remember to look for exit wounds, keeping in mind that it causes a hard impact as well and that you can't predict the path thru the body. We are responding to avenue C and east 10th Street.

Upon arrival on scene we see a young male supine on the sidewalk, a young girl kneeling by him, screaming. I rush to the back of the bus, throwing the trauma gear along with a long board onto the stretcher. As we approach the patient I can see he is breathing. Then I get a little nervous, as I can see a hole right between his eyes. To my surprise there isn't any bleeding.

He is unconscious and his breathing pattern is indicative of some sort of brain injury. We expose him to unsure this is the only injury.

There are a few things that stay constant for every job, no matter what the call. The first priority is the airway, and his is good. Then we go to breathing. Although he is breathing, his breathing pattern is abnormal, so we will have to assist that. My partner has the Ambu-Bag and starts to ventilate him. Needing to be ventilated is bad, and as my partner bags him every push of air into him causes some brain matter to shoot out of the hole between his eyes.

We quickly move him into the ambulance. A breathing tube is placed into the trachea, which stops the brain matter from shooting out of the hole. My partner did that while I prepared to start the IV.

Being a rookie paramedic and my first shooting, I was pretty excited. My adrenalin was pumping as I moved the needle close to the vein in his arm. My hands were shaking so much I could have threaded a sewing machine while it was running.

My experienced partner says to me, "Guy, take it easy. You're not the one who is shot!" Now, that didn't help my ego any but I have to admit, it was funny. Not at the time of course. I'll have to remember that line. One day when I'm working with some rookie medic down the road, I can be the cool old-timer.

Luck will have it, I get the line and we head to the hospital. Seeing the injury even as a new guy I knew that his outcome would not be a good one. He died about 10 minutes after he arrived in the ER. He was a nice-looking kid. He was involved with gangs or drugs maybe both. Such a waste of a young life.

COP SHOT

It was an early September morning around 7:30 a.m. My partner and I had just gotten our coffees. We were parked at 1st Avenue at 20th Street when over the police radio we hear 10-13,10-13, officer shot 1st Avenue and 29th Street. We both throw our coffees out and head up 1st Avenue. As we race up 1st, I was thinking that this will most likely be unfounded.

Two polices cars are right with us as we get closer and more are coming. Within one minute of the call, four police cars and two ambulances are on scene. A basic ambulance was coming out of Bellevue's ER which is right at 26th and 1st Avenue. They are the first to arrive and have started working on the man, who is shot in the chest. He is in traumatic arrest and they are doing CPR.

We assisted the basic unit, they are doing a great job. They have him exposed, are doing CPR and have him placed on long board. We quickly place the endotracheal tube and put in a large bore IV, then we all head to Bellevue's emergency room.

The hospital was on stand by for this officer in traumatic arrest. His wallet was with him showing a small gold shield. We turn him over to the emergency room staff and we watch as they hopelessly try everything they can to save him. They open his chest with the rib spreaders. They can see the heart has a large hole in it from a large caliber bullet. At this point they stop their resuscitative efforts.

Nothing more can be done for him. However, as we start to try to get his identification things are not all as they seem. The wallet with the shield is the wallet of an FBI agent. The picture is not of the dead man on the gurney. As a little more time passes, police and FBI agents come into the trauma slot. Now we get to hear what really happened.

The dead man on the gurney was a man who robed the FBI agent while he was on a stakeout on 29th Street. He had walked up to the parked car, putting a gun to the agent's head and demanding his wallet, which the agent gave him.

Then the robber walked down 29th Street. The agent got out of his vehicle and yelled, "Halt! Police!" The robber fired a shot at the agent, missing him. The agent returned fire, not missing and striking him directly in the heart, as we got to see after they opened his chest. The agent went somewhere and was not on scene, so when people saw the police shield they thought it was that of the man who had been shot. That was why it was called in as cop shot.

It was a pretty interesting call to start the day. We joked about the fact that if you are going to be a bad guy you should be sure to know who your victims are. Picking an FBI agent as a victim was a poor choice. He won't make that mistake again.

THE POOL HALL SHOOTING

It was a quiet Sunday evening one summer. We had just completed a job to Bellevue hospital for something uneventful. As we headed back to our area the police radio broke the silence.

"Robbery squad to central with a priority." In a calm voice the officer reports, "Shots fired, numerous shots fired, from vehicle in front of us into the pool hall on 12th Street between 4th and 5th Avenue. The description of vehicle is a black Nissan, three Asian males are the occupants. Request backup, we are following them. We are in unmarked blue Ford sedan. We are east-bound on 12th Street passing 3rd Avenue at this time."

The next thing we hear are numerous police units saying that they are responding to assist. Cops are heading from all directions: 13th Precinct, 9th Precinct, and ESU units are all racing to join the unmarked robbery unit.

In a short time the guys in the Nissan realize the police are after them. They stop the car and start running on foot in different directions. This was scary to hear, as we were listening to the officers now chasing after these men with guns. It was unbelievable but within a few minutes they were able to catch all three without a single shot being fired.

A great job by the police units and I still can't get over how calm the robbery squad cop was that made the call. Picture yourself seeing guys with guns shooting, being right there and that you are going to have to try to stop them. Your heart would be racing, your mouth dry. This guy sounded like he was saying he was going for fuel.

Anyway, let's see what happened at the pool hall where all those shots were fired. As this police activity was going on my partner and I started to head toward the pool hall just in case someone was hit by one of the many bullets. Over the EMS. radio, a basic unit had also heard about the shots fired and was only a few blocks away and told the dispatcher they would check to see if an ambulance was needed there.

After about a minute that unit was on scene. This time the message that came over the air was not in a calm manner but was very frantic. "Central,

BY NEW YORK CITY PARAMEDIC GEORGE STEFFENSEN

we have five confirmed shot. All serious. Send us backup."

I was driving and took off towards the pool hall. We advised the dispatcher we were a minute out. Over the EMS radio we could hear the other units responding too. This sure changed a slow Sunday evening into a job to remember. The good news was that there were all these units available; two of our medic units, two medic units from St Vincent's Hospital and one medic unit from Bellevue Hospital. All five guys that were shot were in serious condition. One died in the hospital, the other four did well and would get discharged after some time in the hospital. This shooting was gang related.

SPRING STREET

One evening we were dispatched to a shooting on Spring Street in the lobby of the building. As we got out of the ambulance I could see a man on the floor of the lobby. It was just our unit on scene; the police had not arrived yet.

When we got inside, the man said, "I've been shot and can't breathe." I can see that a bullet had entered his forehead, gone around the skull and exited out the front of his neck. Looking closely, his trachea appears intact so I don't understand why he has trouble breathing. He is alert and nervous, but then who wouldn't be after being shot in the head?

I reassure him that we are going to help him and that he has to do what we say. We hold inline stabilization and lay him down on the long board. Then we start to cut away his clothes to see if he has any other injuries.

Boy, does he, and now I understand why he is having trouble breathing. This guy is shot several times in the chest and a few times in the arms. Don't forget the one to his head that comes out his neck. When we are done counting he has a total of twelve bullet holes in him.

Surprising to me and anyone else there isn't much blood, and so far his vital signs are good. Let's not be crazy though, this guy is extremely lucky to be alive and these injuries are life threatening.

Keeping things in right order, one: the airway is intact and patent. The breathing is a problem. The holes in the chest affect his breathing as air is leaking from the holes. We seal them up with occlusive dressing, watching that his condition doesn't worsen due to a tension pneumothorax.

Quickly we move him to the bus; the IVs will be done en route to the hospital. On the way, I ask him if he knew who did it. What the hell was I thinking? Lucky for me he said he didn't know. Like, what would I do if he said some name like John you-know-who. Well he didn't know (good thing for me) but after the fact I remember I'm a medic, not a cop.

He remains conscious when we arrive at the trauma center, but his pulse is rising and his blood pressure is dropping. This happens to be a very bad sign. They decide to take him straight up to the operating room. I hear over the speakers in the emergency room, "Trauma team code blue repeat trauma team code blue." Usually a trauma case will get worked up in the trauma room. When it is a case like this, immediate surgery is the best choice of action. The code blue is the hospital signal for the trauma team to report directly to the operating room.

They work on him for several hours but the injuries are far too great. He does not make it.

JUMPERS

The jumper calls that I have responded to fall pretty much into two types. The jumper up is the jumper who is on a roof, ledge or windowsill with the potential of jumping or falling. As long as they are the jumper up, there isn't much a medic needs to do. Most of the time the police are able to talk the person into not jumping.

They will then give us the patient, and we will evaluate and examine him or her to be sure the irrational behavior is not from a medical condition or drug induced. We will treat any condition as needed. If it is just a psychiatric problem we will keep the patient safe and transport to the emergency room.

Then you have the jumper down. This too has two different types. The jumper who has jumped or fallen from a very high place; he will be dead and again not much for the medic to do there. You will go over to this patient and confirm that they are not alive; in most cases where they have fallen over ten stories this will not be hard to determine. Then finally you have the jumper who has jumped or fallen from a high place and is injured. Now this is a patient that the paramedic will be able to do something for. Finally, a call where we can put all this medic training to use. I will tell you some of my jumper stories.

BY NEW YORK CITY PARAMEDIC GEORGE STEFFENSEN

MY FIRST JUMPER

As a rookie medic, we were dispatched to a jumper down behind a building on the Bowery. We had been to this building in the past, it was a homeless shelter for men. Being new and never seeing a jumper down before I was a little nervous. I was worried about how bad it could be and wondered how I would handle seeing something like this. Besides worrying about that, I was also going over my trauma protocols. I remember thinking whatever you do, do not faint.

As we pulled up on scene we got out of the ambulance and grabbed our long board, c-collar, trauma bag and oxygen. We headed toward the back where a worker had directed us to go. As we approached where the patient was, a cop from around the corner warned us to be careful. "Be careful when you get closer that you don't step on any brains," he yelled to us. Right away I knew from that bit of information that this will be a call that won't be too hard to determine if the patient is alive or dead. The next thing I'm thinking is, how awful is this going to be. I took a deep breath and continued toward the patient. In front of me is a man who jumped about six stories and landed directly on his head. It split open much like a melon. His face was distorted and an eye had popped out. Part of his brains had come out some too .It was hard to look at and at the same time hard to look away. Looking closer, I notice that his arms are both broken and his leg is broken too. It is so strange to see that, my mind was trying to take all in. This is of course obvious death, not much for us to do but to get some information.

My partner, with the help of the police on scene, finds some identification for this man. He writes down the information to fill out our ambulance call report. Then we put our equipment away and get ready for another call.

I will think about this job most of the night and my mind will play back how strange it all looked. I feel bad for this guy and wonder what was so bad that he would end his life. He picked a tough way to do it too.

Over the years more calls like this will come and go. With time, and without realizing it, I will develop a way of not remembering how awful the things I just saw were. It must be some sort of protection mechanism for workers that deal with these kinds of stresses. You are not aware of the slow changes, but they come. It is a way to save yourself, so you may continue to do your job.

BROOKLYN BRIDGE

It was a cold night in December, about 9:00 p.m. I had been a medic awhile when I did this one. We were called to the Brooklyn Bridge for the jumper up. As we pulled next to the East River, just under the bridge we saw police harbor units. ESU Truck One and the two smaller units pull near our ambulance. The police from the ESU truck were putting on their dive gear, ready to go into the water if the jumper does in fact jump into the river. A police helicopter is above with his searchlight scanning the bridge, looking for the jumper.

Sure enough, there is a man high up on the bridge. He is above the roadway of the bridge and has climbed up on some of the support cables. Other police officers are seen on the bridge heading towards the man. When they start to get a little closer the man jumps.

Some things to think about here: first, he jumped from very high up. Then he is jumping into icy waters. And the East River is not very clean. I forgot to mention that this is a black man dressed in all black. I did mention that it was 9:00 p.m.

Well, the harbor unit (along with the divers) jumps into the water in their dry dive suits to search for him. Unbelievable as it is, the guy pops up out of the water pretty close to the harbor boat. Within a few minutes the harbor guys and the divers are pulling him out of the water. The ESU officers place a c-collar and long board onto the patient and get his pulse.

The patient is stable and only complains of back soreness. This was truly a small miracle. The harbor unit brings him to the closest dock and transfers him to our ambulance, where we reevaluate him. He is in good shape; he has tried in the past to hurt himself. I guess he will have to try again another time. Someone up there is watching out for him. His vital signs are good, no obvious signs of injury.

We take him to the emergency room where he gets transferred over to the psychiatric ward for further evaluation. Cops from Brooklyn came to the emergency ward just to see the guy, as they can't believe he survived this jump.

BY NEW YORK CITY PARAMEDIC GEORGE STEFFENSEN

SOUTH STREET

It was about 6:00 p.m. when we were dispatched to 180 South Street for the jumper up. As we pull in front of the building we see a man on the ledge of the roof. The roof has a fence around the edges and he has climbed over this protective railing. The building is 20 stories tall. Another ambulance pulls in behind our unit and a number of police units have arrived on scene too.

We pull our equipment out of the ambulance; I guess more for show because if he jumps from 20 stories we won't be taking him. My partner has been on the job a long time so I follow his lead and know that what he is doing will keep us from getting into trouble.

The jumper is walking along the edge and not only am I worried that he might jump, but also that he could just as easily slip and fall by accident. The next minutes seem like a lifetime as we see him so close to the edge. The police are making their way up to the rooftop so they can try to talk him down as they have done many times in the past in similar situations.

They have made it onto the roof now. The man sees them as he is holding the railing. He drops down and is now just holding on with his hands. While he hangs there for a moment there is not a sound to be heard. Everyone is looking in disbelief hoping that he will not let himself go. I wonder if he has the strength to pull himself up. The police try to get to him to pull him back up.

He starts to pull himself up but in the same motion he pulls up and pushes himself away from the building, letting go. As he is falling part of me wants to turn away. I watch, as I guess I'm mesmerized by this unusual event. There isn't a sound until we hear the thud of his body hitting the ground. He bounces up about 6 feet and then lands again, this time motionless.

Over a radio I hear someone screaming he's down, he's down, he's down. We quickly run over to where his lifeless body is, to confirm the obvious. It was very strange, but to see him lying there, you would not have guessed he just fell 20 stories. It wasn't the mess you would expect.

He landed on a grassy area. We were lucky that he missed the metal railing, which was around the grass. Watching someone jump 20 stories was something that still stays in my mind. We stayed on the scene and when the police were done we helped the basic unit remove the body. Although he didn't look so bad, when we moving him you could feel his body and realize the amount of broken bones he had sustained, along with the other internal injuries.

Jumping like that, having all that time on the way down…how awful it must be. Hell, it was tough on me just watching. People have so many problems. When I see how bad things for others are it reminds me how small my problems are and truly how lucky I am.

DUMB CRIMINAL

This story lets you understand that criminals are not the brightest. We get dispatched to the jumper down on 9th Street and Avenue C. We arrive on scene as the police pull up with us. We are directed to the alley where a man has fallen or jumped from about six stories. We bring our stretcher, long board and the rest of our trauma equipment to the alley for the man down. As we quickly check the patient, we easily determine that he is dead. Obvious death, so we will not need to work him up.

However, while we are examining him we notice that he has a thin rope under his arms somewhat the size of a clothes line. The police are talking to another man who is very distressed. He is telling the police that the man fell from the roof. The cop asks, "What were you doing up on the roof?" The man hesitates but then confesses to the fact they were up there and were going to rob the apartment below on the fifth floor. The plan was that he was going to lower him from the roof with his thin rope to the 5th floor open window.

The robber climbed over the ledge with his friend holding the rope. He had tied the end of the rope to a pipe to help him, a safety precaution. After a very short time the rope broke, unable to hold his weight. His friend quickly fell the six stories to the pavement between the buildings. You have to wonder how that, between the two of these grown men, they couldn't figure out that a clothesline wouldn't be the best choice of equipment to use. Unfortunately, they took a chance and it cost this man his life. The other thing I think about was, what great valuables were they going to find in this project apartment that would be worth risking going to jail, much less risking their lives over? Well it happened, people do crazy things for reasons we can't understand.

BY NEW YORK CITY PARAMEDIC GEORGE STEFFENSEN

CONSTRUCTION WORKER

I am working with big Andy Mazzola when we are dispatched to a jumper down at a construction site at East 25th Street and Lexington Avenue. As we get on scene we can see a building in the early stages of construction. Mostly the only part of the building that is up is the steel frame. There is some flooring but it looks incomplete and temporary.

A construction worker runs over to us and points up at the building telling us that one of the steel workers fell from the ninth floor beams and landed on some temporary flooring on the seventh floor.

Andy and I get our trauma equipment and head up to the patient. It is difficult getting to him. There are a lot of beams and other construction materials we have to climb by to get up the seven stories. When we finally get to the patient, he is lying on his back, awake but being very still.

I'm not checking the patient as much as I am looking at the temporary floor I'm standing on. It doesn't look very safe. I can see the dent the patient made in it from his fall. I can also see the ground through the gaps and I'm not so good with heights.

Getting back to the patient, I start doing the physical exam. Andy gets information from the patient as to what happened and what complaints he has.

At first glance I notice a big steel wrench going right through his lower arm. It isn't bleeding much and I ask him if there is anything else hurting him besides the obvious arm problem. He tells me that his back hurts a little but his main complaint is definitely the arm with the big wrench sticking through it.

After doing a head-to-toe exam and getting his vital signs, we consider him to be a stable patient. I explain to him because he fell and has back pain we will be placing him on a long board and putting a collar on him as a precaution. Removing him from this dangerous position is going to be a little complicated. He is in a lot of pain and I get orders for morphine. By this time cops from the emergency service unit have joined us on the seventh floor.

While I get the IV in place and give him some morphine to ease the pain. Andy immobilizes his lower arm to keep the big wrench from moving and causing further damage.

Being busy and focused on the patient, I was less nervous. However, once I am done pushing the morphine I look down, scaring myself again. I tell myself to stay focused of the patient and I'll be all right.

The emergency services cops working with the construction crew figured the easiest way to get him safely to the ground while being on the long board will be to be lower him with the crane. The ESU cops have their Stokes basket brought up with the crane in a big construction box. It is big enough to hold the Stokes basket and two men.

We place the patient into the Stokes basket and I ask him how he was doing. He tells me, "The morphine really has helped!" I smile as I see the morphine is doing its job. I reassess his vital signs and assure him he will be all right. We prepare to go up in the crane. I ride in the box with the patient and one of the ESU cops.

As the big box swings away from the building I have a great view of the street way below. Looking down I see lots of people looking up pointing at us as we make our way down. The closer we get to the ground, the better I feel. We get down and Andy is there with the stretcher.

We load the patient into the ambulance and take him over to the hospital. His x-ray shows the wrench nicely through the lower arm between the two bones. He was very lucky that there were no fractures and that it also missed any major veins or arteries.

That was an exciting job, being up there and getting to ride in the crane; something we don't do every day. The patient was very nice too and he had a great outcome.

A few months later, Andy Mazzola and I received medals for bravery for this dangerous job. Something else that doesn't happen often.

PIN JOBS

THE ROLL OVER

It was a summer afternoon when I was working upstate in Rockland. We were just driving around when the dispatcher gave us a job for a rollover. A car had flipped over at a small side street location.

As we started in that direction a police car that was coming on scene saw the overturned vehicle and right away requested the medics to step it up. This confirmed that the call was real. Then just as quickly the cop said to advise the medics to slow it down. So we start to slow it down a little, and then the cop is saying have the medics step it up again. What the heck is going on? we thought.

We arrive on scene to see a young man standing with minor lacerations to his face. The car is still on its roof. He doesn't look that bad. So this was why we got the slow down.

Then the cop quickly yells he's fine but there is a guy trapped under the car, it's his brother. Well this explains why we got the step it up again. Looking at the back of the car the roof and rear trunk are touching the ground. Between the spaces where the rear window and the ground meet there is a gap. In that small space I see a pair of legs sticking out from under the car.

At first, I thought that I was looking at someone who has been crushed to death. I rush over to him and slide under to see if he is alive and conscious. To my surprise and his luck he is very much alive and tells me that his ass hurts.

I tell him to lie still, that the fire department is coming and we will get him out from under the car. The firefighters arrive and, using air bags, are able to raise the car so that we can immobilize him and get him out from underneath. Once out from that predicament we are able to do a complete head to toe evaluation.

He was extremely lucky. His only real injury was a very big laceration to his butt. He was the passenger and when the car flipped he was thrown half way out the rear window, landing in the small void between the roof and the trunk. His brother was so relieved that he was going to be all right except for the extra crack in his ass.

TRUCK INTO THE TREE

On one early morning, again working up in Rockland, we were en route to a difficulty breathing call. We were just cancelled from that job. As soon as we were cancelled we heard over the police scanner they were in pursuit of a pick-up truck. They were traveling at a high rate of speed down some winding roads.

The pick up truck lost control crashing in to a big tree. The driver jumped out, leaving the scene. There was another young man inside the truck. He struck the windshield and was knocked unconscious. Seeing lots of blood coming from his head the police request an ambulance. "Have the medics step it up," we hear over the radio.

We were only three blocks from the call and arrived on scene within two minutes. Getting out of our unit I see the police at the passenger door working hard to open it. Smoke and flames are coming from the engine compartment. The passenger door is damaged from the impact and two cops work hard with some pry bar in an attempt to get access to the unconscious man.

I rush over to the driver's side of the truck. This door opens easily. I'm going to be the hero and pull the unconscious man out of the burning truck, of course maintaining inline stabilization. At this point I'm feeling the heat and the smoke is starting to make me cough. I grab the man and try to pull him to safety. He starts to slide across the seat but then I can't move him.

Then I see his leg is pinned. His foot is crushed by the door and it is holding him in the truck. More police units have arrived on scene they are all using their small fire extinguishers in efforts to quell the fire. Things don't look good. The smoke and flames are too close to me and the patient. Something has to change and very quick.

While the cops are trying to knock down the fire I place an IV into the unconscious man. He is breathing, we have already placed a c-collar on him and his vitals are good.

We need to get him out as the fire is getting bigger and the heat and smoke are worse. Thoughts are going through my head now: I'm not going to watch this guy burn to death. Now believe it or not, I have a plan.

In the next few minutes things change for the better. Fire trucks pull up and in no time the fire and smoke are not an issue any longer. I am so relieved.

Once the fire is knocked down, other firemen use the Jaws of Life and free his foot. We are now able to immobilize his injuries and we have him in the ambulance.

He starts to come around. He has a big laceration to the face and a broken foot but he will be all right in a few weeks.

As for his friend who left him to die in the burning truck, I never found out if they ever caught him.

Oh, my plan. I forgot to tell you my plan. The truth is I don't know if I could have done it. Watching a guy burn to death was not going to happen. Life over limb, the plan was to cut his foot off. Thank God we will never know that, if things didn't go the way they did, would I have been able to do it?

One thing for sure, I would have had some explaining to do at call review. I've worked in a lot of areas and so far I haven't seen the amputation protocol.

THE STUCK HAND

Here I am on the lower east side when we get the call for the confirmed pin job. It is a young man who was working the trash compactor. While pushing some garbage into the compactor it closed on his hand, crushing it and trapping his arm in the machine.

He was in a lot of pain. His vitals were good. It was an isolated injury so as they worked to free him we were able to get orders for morphine to relieve some of the pain. We were there on scene a long time as the emergency service cops worked to free him. The morphine helped take some of the pain away but you could see he was afraid of what was happening to him. We knew that his hand was crushed to the point that he would surely loose it. Sad for this young working guy.

Things were not going well for the cops either. They had been working for over an hour and they weren't making much progress. The emergency service sergeant came over to us. "We're having trouble, I think you should call for a physician to come and amputate his hand."

Now this is a request you don't get very often. Funny, last job I was telling you I was thinking of cutting off the guy's foot and here the cop wants to have a doctor cut his hand off. Goes to show you my plan wasn't that crazy.

I call telemetry, they are the doctors that give us our orders. We advise them of the situation. After being placed on hold for a while, they advise me that an EMS supervisor and a doctor with amputation equipment are en route to our location. Just as the physician and supervisor arrive on scene the young man's badly crushed hand is freed from the compactor. We wrap it up and take him over to the hospital. The trauma team takes a look at his badly crushed hand and preps him to go to the operating room. I'm afraid my evaluation of the injury was correct and they will have to amputate his hand.

BY NEW YORK CITY PARAMEDIC GEORGE STEFFENSEN

MOTORCYCLE DOWN

It was a nice summer afternoon and my partner and I were parked at St Marks and 2nd Avenue. Over the police radio we hear a cop calling for a bus forthwith, motorcyclist struck by a cab. He requests emergency service units as well.

The motorcyclist is pinned under the taxi. The call is on 14th Street and Avenue C. Our unit advises the EMS dispatcher of the job on 14 and C and we are only one minute out. As we grab our trauma equipment and run over to the cab I see the fire engine racing towards us.

We see the motorcyclist is pinned under the cab and he is in traumatic cardiac arrest. We can't get to his head to attempt to open his airway. I'm glad that the engine company is right there; time is critical. Without an airway he has no chance. I tell the firemen that he is pinned and we need them to lift the car off him with their air bags. The firemen tell me that the engines don't have the airbags but a ladder truck is in route. Just as he tells me that, Truck One from police emergency service units are pulling on scene. The car is off him in seconds. I go for the intubation as my partner gets the IV lines in place. The firemen from the engine are assisting us with the CPR. His airway is full of blood and intubation is nearly impossible. I blindly pass the tube through the blood. I know that this guy is dead; he is not going to survive this hit. Still, I want to get the tube. I did get it and we quickly get him into the bus. We are off the scene in about 15 minutes and, being a pin job and having to wait until we could get him from under the car, it was pretty quick. The hospital is just three minutes away. We have him in the trauma slot; we give the report.

The doctors try their best but really, this will be more like practice for the interns, as he really doesn't have a chance. From a technical point we did a good job. Police, Fire, and EMS, we all worked well together. The sad thing is this young motorcycle guy is dead because the cab that he went under was making an illegal U-turn. I know that having the interns doing a lot of the work might not seem like the right thing to do, but they need to get the hands-on experience. Another day, that extra experience might help the doctor do something in a more timely fashion. Which might make the difference for someone else.

MY FIRST YEAR IN THE CITY

I started working in the city after being a paramedic for about two years. I still have a lot to learn. The paramedics in Rockland and Westchester have helped me a lot. However, the call volume was low and I still need more experience to know what I am doing.

The city is so different from where I grew up. The area that I am working is the lower east side. This area has lots of homeless people. Tompkins Square Park is full of all kinds of people who are on drugs or drunk. Shootings and stabbings around here are not unusual. Heroin is a big problem at this time. I can't believe how many overdoses I handle in just one tour. Doing three heroin overdoses in an eight-hour tour was a routine day. Hell, one day I basically save one guy twice in one tour. First I picked him up at about 8:00 a.m. He was blue, his respiratory rate was about four per minute and he was on the verge of going into cardiac arrest. We shoot him with two milligrams of Narcan and he is fine. He stays in the emergency room for three hours and leaves. About an hour late I get another call for him! The same exact situation; he was blue, slow respirations and again on the verge of cardiac arrest. We give him the two of Narcan and back to the hospital.

I'm very excited about working here in the big city. To me this is the big league. I still work part time up in Westchester and Rockland and I love telling the others that I'm a medic in the city. I don't tell them how nervous I am or how the senior medics let me know I'm a rookie. To the city medics, working in Westchester and Rockland was nothing, only time as a city medic counted. In my defense, people's anatomy is the same whether up in the country or in a big city, but I'll keep that comment to myself. I will admit that I was intimidated when patients who were on drugs or drunk would get violent. Trying to deal with junkies and people who are drunk, there is no reasoning with them. Most of the time in order for you to get them into the ambulance or onto the stretcher you will have to physically put them there. I was very scared that they might hurt me. Using force on someone was new to me and these people were tough, and I am not. My thoughts are that I'm a nice guy trying to help you, why would you try to hurt me?

Being a relatively new paramedic I was eager to buff calls. I was always listening to both the police and the emergency medical radio. Ready to chase after any call that sounds like something good. I still carry all my equipment like the rookie medic I am. Still going over the protocols in my mind as we rush to the different assignments. Thinking (or more hoping, I guess) that at the calls we are dispatched to I will be able to use my training and maybe save a life.

HOMELESS PEOPLE

When I first started working in the city it was a new experience for me to be directly involved with homeless people. I grew up in Westchester County, Chappaqua, New York to be exact. This is where President Clinton now resides. Seeing people living on the streets was something that I was not familiar with. This will of course change over time. I will get the chance to be very familiar with a number of homeless people and get the opportunity to see a different way of life that I will never understand. Let me take you to the streets and I will share with you some of my experiences with these special people.

The first homeless guy I can remember was George. We were dispatched to 10th Street and Avenue C. There, lying on the sidewalk was an older man about fifty. He was very dirty and his pants were soaked with urine. He had been drinking and was complaining that his back hurt. He spoke to us in a very demanding way and he looked pretty big. His hands were big and rough from being on the streets. I was intimidated by him.

New here in the city and dealing with this mean, homeless guy, I felt way out of my element. I wasn't really sure how to handle this kind of call. This stuff is not taught in the books or the classroom. I nervously tell him I am here to help him. He yells at me to put him on the stretcher. He keeps grabbing his back screaming at us to help. We carefully pick him up and place him onto the stretcher. As we lift the stretcher into the ambulance a huge fist swings past my face, just missing me. This was certainly something that I didn't expect. Although I am scared and not sure what to do I have to do something to gain control of this situation. I feel I have an advantage as he is lying on the stretcher. As soon as the stretcher is in the ambulance I jump on top of him and my partner joins in. We quickly subdue him and restrain him by tying him to the stretcher, to protect him and us from possible injury.

"What are you doing trying to hit me? I'm here helping you," I said as I catch my breath. He starts to say something but his words are so slurred that it is hard to understand what he is saying. At this point what he has to say is not important. If he is well enough to take a swing at me for no reason he'll be fine until we reach the hospital. One thing I do know, if you have to restrain someone they stay that way until we are at the hospital and security can worry about untying them.

Well I'm not in Chappaqua anymore, that's for sure. My first dealings with a homeless guy and he almost cleaned my clock. If that big fist connected I'm sure I would have been knocked out. How embarrassing that would have been. Here I am dealing with my first homeless drunk and he knocks me out. It would have been a very bad start. I'm sure to this day everyone still would be making fun of the rookie medic who got knocked out by the drunk. Lucky for me, that wasn't the case. This is a good lesson for me and I'll keep in mind what this guy looks like if I should ever get sent to him again.

I will get to pick up George on lots of occasions over the years. I will learn later that he is an ex-Marine and a combat veteran. He will, on some of his more lucid days, share some stories and tell me about his experiences in Vietnam. He tells me that he served at the same time as my brother and that he had received the silver star medal.

He still will keep on drinking and will not hesitate to take a swing at me even though we have a strange bond. I think he has mental problems besides his drinking problem. I say this, as he starts these fights knowing full well that he will be on the losing end. I worry about him; I know he has been through a lot so I do my best to help this fellow Marine. On the good days when I have to pick him up, we get along and he is amusing. I could do a whole book on my homeless buddies, but let me get this one done first.

One more quick George story. A fancy hospital north of Bellevue Hospital opened up its emergency room to the 911 system. Prior to that it mostly received private patients in its emergency room. Certainly, it did not know what this would mean to the emergency room staff. It will now be getting a lot of homeless drunks from the nearby men's shelter. It will also be getting loads of the patients who pretend to be sick to get food and shelter on cold nights. They were not very happy with the ambulance crews who started to bring in these new "patients."

I think we all got off on the wrong foot. Things are good between the crews and the emergency room staff now. It was that adjustment period that things were a little hard.

One night during this "adjustment period" I was sent to Avenue C and 9th Street for guess who? Very good; you're right, George. It was about 10:00 p.m. and I had an hour before getting off. We needed to waste some time. What's wrong tonight I ask George. He says honestly, "I just want some food and to get into a bed." I was surprised by his answer. He must not be feeling up to playing tonight.

I tell him about this new emergency room that opened. I wink and tell him "Georgie, they don't know you like the rest of the emergency rooms do. You tell them you have chest pain and they will keep you overnight for sure."

He likes the idea and shakes his head yes with approval. "All right Georgie, get on the stretcher." We work him up just like a real cardiac patient. We put oxygen on him. We do an electrocardiogram. We place an intravenous line in him. At least he looks like a cardiac patient. Now he is ready for his trip to the fancy emergency room. We give him an aspirin too. This is like the cherry on an ice cream Sunday. Giving him nitro for the "chest pain" would be taking it a bit too far. Plus we can get past that by telling them the pain was gone on our arrival. We advise George to say he had chest pain but that the pain is gone now. Certainly an aspirin will not hurt anyone. Of course we checked that he has no allergies. We don't want anything bad to happen to our buddy.

We bring George into the emergency room and tell our story about this man with chest pain. His clothes are not clean but you would not think he was homeless. After the nurse is done with us we place George on the emergency stretcher the nurse starts asking her questions.

"Sir what was the pain like on a scale of one to ten?" I put up seven fingers behind her and George quickly says seven. "Do you have trouble breathing?" the nurse asks. George's eyes look to me. I shake my head yes. George replies, "Yes." "Any nausea?" Again my head shakes yes and George responds accordingly. Next question, "Does the pain go anywhere?" Again my head shakes a positive yes as I rub my jaw. George again comes through. "Yes, I have pain to my jaw!" George states very convincingly. Hell, for a moment even I thought George was having a heart attack.

BY NEW YORK CITY PARAMEDIC GEORGE STEFFENSEN

Well there you go, George was admitted for observation. The good news is all the tests and lab work will come back just fine. Not surprising to us of course. George will be back out on the streets in a few days.

ROBERT

Another favorite homeless guy was this big man named Robert. When I first started picking him up I was very intimidated by him. I've said before that I'm pretty big, but Robert was almost as tall as I am and he was very muscular. Someone that I would not want to fight. He was more of a happy drunk. I was always careful not to do anything to change that.

His trademark expression whenever we picked him up was to say "I'm not black I'm cocoa brown." He was always messing around with the crews. When you would catch him sober he was really very pleasant. He would be sure to thank you for the many times you had helped him.

Sadly, I must say that Robert was the homeless man we lost on that cold winter's night. Lots of us that had the pleasure of picking up our friend who was "not black but cocoa brown" will always remember Robert.

BY NEW YORK CITY PARAMEDIC GEORGE STEFFENSEN

MY JACK NICHOLSON IMITATION

We are in the business of saving lives, and while my existence to you may be grotesque, we save lives.

Son we live in a world where there are ambulances, and on these ambulances there are medics. Are you going to do it. We use words like defibrillate, intubate, cardiovert, we use them as a way of saving lives. You people use them after you have seen Third Watch.

I have neither the time nor the inclination to explain myself to someone who calls an ambulance and then questions the manner in which I provide it. I would rather you just say thank you and be on your way. Otherwise I suggest you grab a defibrillator and get on a bus. Either way I don't give a damn what you think you are entitled to.

About this book, on the record I tell you that anything inappropriate or out of protocol never happened, it was just to make it more interesting. Off the record I tell you the stuff is unbelievable and if it was done without my supervisor's knowledge then so be it.

If you want to investigate me, roll the dice and take your chances. I eat breakfast 300 yards from Alphabet City and believe me, that's dangerous. So don't think for one second you can call a supervisor and make me nervous.

So you want an ambulance. I'll give you all the ambulances you want, but first you have to ask me nicely. You see, I can deal with the blood and the guts. I don't want money. I don't want medals. What I do want is for you to stand there in your fancy suit and your Harvard mouth and extend me some fucking courtesy. I want you to ask me nicely!

BY NEW YORK CITY PARAMEDIC GEORGE STEFFENSEN

PEDESTRIANS STRUCK

People get hit by cars everyday. I never realized how often until I started working in the city. Just like any other call, the pedestrian struck can be as simple as a minor injury or as severe as a fatality. I'll start off with a somewhat funny job.

BY NEW YORK CITY PARAMEDIC GEORGE STEFFENSEN

THE LEG JOB

We were dispatched to a pedestrian struck at East 23rd and 3rd Avenue. As we start to the call we hear over the police radio a cop calling his dispatcher to advise EMS to rush the bus, the man down is a heavy bleeder. Our unit is only two blocks away and we are on scene in seconds. A basic unit arrives with us very quickly. The man is on the ground; he was hit by a bus. He has a lot of blood from his legs. He is also unconscious. My partner and I start to check his airway and breathing. I ask the new guy on the basic unit to start to expose him so we can get a better look to see where all this blood is coming from. The EMT is wearing heavy rubber gloves. As he starts to remove the man's shoes he pulls on the man's leg. While he is pulling on the leg, the whole leg starts coming out of the pants. The EMT turns as pale as the patient. As the leg comes fully out of the pants we can see it is an artificial leg. The color starts to come back to the EMT and the rest of us. The patient starts to regain consciousness as we further expose and evaluate him. We find the blood is coming from an open femur fracture on the real leg. His leg was crushed by the bus and this injury is pretty severe. We immobilize him and do the rest of the proper treatment.

To see that leg come out of the pants was freaky. We all thought his leg had been amputated from the accident. The poor guy pulling on the leg; because of the thick gloves he hadn't noticed the leg was artificial. He was also new and I'm sure with his adrenalin pumping he might not have noticed anyway. What a call for him to start off with. I'm sure he will be telling everyone about that one.

Another interesting fact about this call, as we will later learn: he was run over by a bus before and that is how he lost his leg. A sad thing is that the damage to his leg was so severe that he ended up loosing that leg also. What are the chances of being struck by a bus on two different occasions and both would result in the loss of a leg? Unbelievable but very true.

BY NEW YORK CITY PARAMEDIC GEORGE STEFFENSEN

PEDIATRICS

Pediatric calls are the hardest of all calls no matter how long you have been a paramedic. You don't get that many pediatric calls that are true emergencies, thank God.

So you don't have that much experience with them. There is a big difference when you see an adult lying there than when you see a child lying there.

It is a parent's worst nightmare to have your child die or see them severely injured. Even when I was a buff and wanted to use my new skills I never looked forward to this type of call.

Unfortunately, the calls will come; some will die and some will be severely injured. I can't explain the pressure that is on the paramedics that respond to these calls. The scene is so much more intense. Everything seems like a dream, more like a nightmare. You feel like you can't move quickly enough, knowing that seconds count.

Unlike the adult patient, where the drug dosages come to mind like second nature, you have some tough calculations to make as these drugs are given in milligram/kilograms. So with all the stress you are going through you look at the child. You have to guess their weight in pounds and then switch that to kilograms. Then figure out the drug dosage you want to give.

Their small little bodies are so helpless as you try to manage their tiny airways. Trying for intravenous access is hard enough, but these pediatric patients' veins are much smaller and less prominent. Which makes them much harder to get.

You can't help thinking of a child you know, be it your own son or daughter or some loved one around the same age. Picturing them lying there. Fearing that the outcome will not be a good one. These calls, no matter how tough or callous you think you are or have become, will still stress and affect you.

After you complete a job with a child, especially if the outcome isn't a good one, you will replay the call in your mind a thousand times. Wonder-

BY NEW YORK CITY PARAMEDIC GEORGE STEFFENSEN

ing if there was something you could have done differently or better which
might have changed the outcome for the better.

THE HEALTH CLUB

It was a December evening when I was at the base getting my equipment ready. A call came in for an unconscious child at the local health club pool. I was working a fly car unit in Westchester. I took an EMT with me and we raced towards the health club. The dispatcher was trying to get more information about the call. I was hoping that it might be something not too serious, like maybe a seizure.

Then the dispatcher called confirming that CPR is in progress. It's a seven-year-old boy that has been pulled from the pool. I was already driving too fast, fortunately, the health club was close to where we were. We were pulling into the club after we had received the last message from dispatch. We get our equipment and head into the health club where we are directed to the pool area.

I could see two men doing CPR; one is the lifeguard the other is a doctor who had been working out at the club. My partner took over compressions as I hooked up the monitor to see what rhythm he was in. The doctor continued doing the ventilations as we saw on the monitor that the child was in V-fib. I charged the paddles of the defibrillator and got ready to shock the boy. "Clear," I said loudly to ensure that no one was touching him as I pressed the paddles to his chest. I shocked him and then checked to see what rhythm he went into. Hoping that he will covert into a sinus rhythm.

No he does not, even worse, he goes flat line...asystole. He needs drugs, he needs to be intubated. He is dying right now, we need to get the endotracheal tube placed and we need to give drugs. I move to the head and position myself to place the breathing tube. I'm lucky as when I go to place the tube it is easy to place. Of course I ensure it is in by listening to the stomach and then the lung fields. As that is being done CPR is continued. From time to time we stop to check the rhythm. Still no change; flat line.

The doctor checks his left arm looking for a vein to put an IV. Some drugs can be given down the breathing tube so I give him an epi and an atropine down the tube. More CPR and still no change. I look at his right arm for a vein to place an IV and nothing is showing there either. I look at his neck and see a good neck vein, the external jugular vein. I have placed a few IV lines there in the past but never on a kid. I prepare the site using an 18-gauge catheter and I carefully insert it into the vein. The IV is in and now we repeat the epi and atropine, this time in the line.

Technically, the job has been moving forward very well. Early CPR, along with early advanced life support. The initial rhythm was V-fib. Defibrillation was done quickly, breathing tube placed in a timely manner and drugs given per protocol. Unfortunately, this boy is still in cardiac arrest as we load him up to into the ambulance. We give one more epi in the ambulance and do CPR. We stop CPR to check once more to see if there is any change on the monitor.

I can't believe what I see, a nice sinus rhythm at about 100 beats per minute. I know this is just part of the picture; you can have a good rhythm without a pulse. Next I feel for a pulse, and he has a nice one. As we are arriving at the emergency room we find he has a good blood pressure too. The emergency doctors and nursing staff are waiting as we come in. We give our report as to how we found this boy what was done prior to and once we arrived on scene. Later he will be transferred to a hospital that specializes in pediatrics.

After I am able to replace the equipment we had used on the call we head back to the base, feeling good that the call went well and that this boy has a good chance. Time will tell, but he has a lot going for him. Being young with good bystander CPR and having advanced life support right away certainly may have made the difference. When I am alone after the call I find myself crying. Even though the call had gone well I guess the stress was a bit too much. Tears of joy, tears of thanks; thank God that the call went well.

BABY ARREST

Early one morning we had just pulled up to our street location. This is where we wait for calls. Our unit was stationed at St Marks and 2nd Avenue. We get the call for a baby in cardiac arrest. The call is on 9th Street between Avenue D and Avenue C. We are about five blocks away. Over time I learn that most of the cardiac arrest calls for babies will turn out to be a febrile seizures, which is what I hope this will turn out to be. Before I can put the bus in gear a police car goes flying past us. We take off right behind him. He makes a left up Avenue B; we went up to Avenue D to make the left to get to 9th Street. His way was faster and as we pull on scene the officer has met the father. The father handed the officer the lifeless baby boy.

My partner and I get into the back of the ambulance and clear the stretcher. The officer was doing mouth-to-mouth as he brought him to us. My partner was getting the pediatric equipment ready as I started to check the baby. Trying to keep my thoughts on the protocols, my heart is racing. The stress is, again, so great. As I try to open his tiny mouth in an effort to place the breathing tube, the stress is over.

The stress is over as I realize that he has already started to develop rigor mortis and I can't open his mouth. Looking at his tiny lifeless body almost like a little doll. His tiny little fingers.

I feel guilty that I felt relief that it is over and the stress was off me. Certainly I wanted to do anything and everything had he had even the slightest of chances. There was absolutely nothing anyone could do. He had been dead too long.

We learn later that the father woke up and when he tried to wake his son he couldn't and called 911. The baby most likely died of SIDS, a very tragic thing for any parent to go through.

Any time that I have a pediatric call, especially when it turns out bad, I always think of my kids and how lucky I have been. Knock on wood, that they should stay safe and healthy.

BY NEW YORK CITY PARAMEDIC GEORGE STEFFENSEN

CHILD NOT BREATHING

March 8th, 6:00 a.m. I remember the date, as it is my birthday. I was just about to get off from the overnight shift (my tour ends at 7:00 a.m.) when a call comes in for a child not breathing. Of course my first thoughts again will go to the seizure. More than ninety percent of the arrest calls or not breathing calls will not be anything serious. Rather then write numerous calls about going to the kid that turns out to be just a new mom that got scared her baby wasn't breathing for a second, I will keep the book to what I hope will be more interesting. Let's continue.

I check the map to find the street and get into the fly car, again I am up in Westchester. I'm solo this time and the local volunteer ambulance will be responding too. It takes me about three minutes to get to the house where I see two police cars on scene. I get my equipment and run up to the front door. Just to tell, you when you are alone all that equipment is very heavy. I have the oxygen bag, monitor, and the drug box; it comes close to 80 lbs.

The door is open and a scared mother is pointing up the stairs. In front of me at the top of the stairs are two cops working on a ten-year-old boy whose face is blue from lack of oxygen. They advise me that when they arrived, the boy's twelve-year-old sister had kept him alive by doing mouth-to-mouth on him. There are so many people out there that do great things, this kid's sister certainly did a good job. By giving him mouth-to-mouth before we arrived gave him a better chance. The boy is unconscious and blue as the police try to get air into him with great difficulty. The good news is that he still has a good pulse but he is definitely in very serious condition.

There is no doubt in my mind that if we can't get his breathing improved he will surely die. My thoughts are why is this kid blue, what medical condition does he have that could cause this healthy looking kid to be at death's door. I call to the mother as I get ready to place the breathing tube into him. "Does he have any medical problems?" She says no. "On any medications for anything?" No again. What the hell is going on with this kid? Well, I'm no doctor, but when you don't know what you are treating you go with the basics. First: the airway. He seems to have that; we'll know better when I place the breathing tube. The boy is unconscious at this point. When I open the mouth and put in the laryngoscope I can see the opening to the trachea. There is nothing in there blocking his airway so I place the breathing tube. I check to be sure it is properly placed. First I listen to his stomach. Nothing heard there, so then up to both lungs. Here I can hear lung sounds as I ventilated him. They are equal, so this is where the tube belongs. I tape it in place to keep it from coming out.

We now have the airway taken care of; the next thing is the breathing. Well, his color was blue, so breathing needs to be assisted. Using the Ambu-Bag, we ventilate him. After a minute of assisting his breathing his color improves. His pulse has remained at about 100, which is a good sign. When someone is not breathing, the pulse sometimes slows to dangerous levels and they go into complete cardiac arrest if not corrected in time. So far, things are getting better. As I am placing the breathing tube the ambulance arrives. I tell the crew to set the stretcher up downstairs.

Once they are set up I pick up the boy and carry him down the stairs. Jennifer, an emergency medical technician, ventilates him as we come down to the stretcher. We then place him quickly on the stretcher and get him into the ambulance. We are not going to mess with success; an IV is started en route to the hospital.

We do this so if something else happens and we need to administer drugs we have access to do it. On the way the boy starts to come around; he cannot speak as he has the breathing tube in place.

I say to him, "You can't speak because the tube is there to help you breath. Just shake your head yes or no." I ask him, "Were you eating anything or did anything get stuck in your throat when this happened?" He shook his head no. Still, I have no idea what caused this healthy-looking boy to almost stop breathing. I could see by his eyes opened so wide he was terrified. I tried to let him know that he was doing better. "The emergency room is waiting for us, you'll be okay," I told him.

Later we will find that he had a tumor in his chest near the throat that had obstructed the airway. With the breathing tube in place it was able to get the oxygen into his lungs past the tumor. This boy had many operations to remove the tumor. For many years (eight, as a matter of fact) I would get cards from him and his family.

He had some good years; he went through a lot. He finished high school and was going to college. Unfortunately, as I would do at Christmas, I sent them Christmas cards but this year I didn't receive one back. I thought maybe they had moved. Around New Year's I received a letter from them saying that this year they didn't send out cards. They weren't celebrating this year, the year that their son had more cancer and had died very unexpectedly just before Christmas.

This was a very sad day to learn he had died. Thanks to his sister and with our help he was able to have eight more years with his family.

This is a call that will always stay with me. I will always remember him and his family. Always remember the cards they took the time to write on our special day, March 8th, and the Christmas cards too.

BY NEW YORK CITY PARAMEDIC GEORGE STEFFENSEN

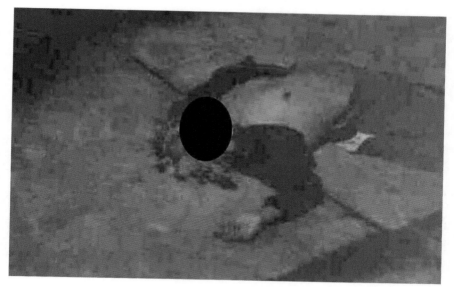

1st Jumper down.

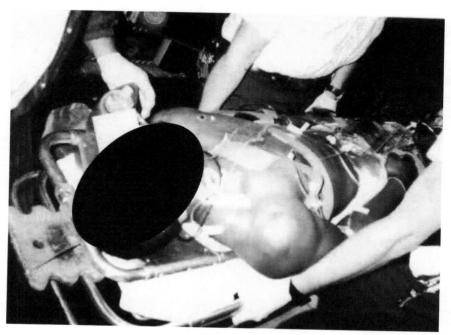

Gun shot wound to chest

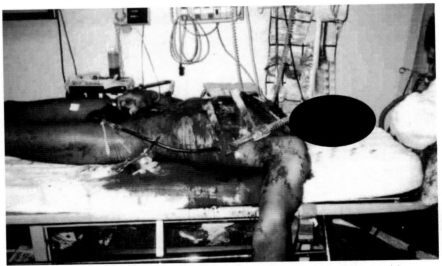

Gun shot wound to chest after they have stopped working on him.

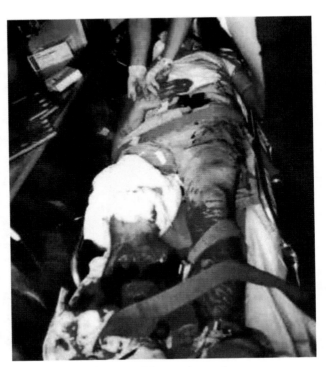

Shot gun blast to lower leg.

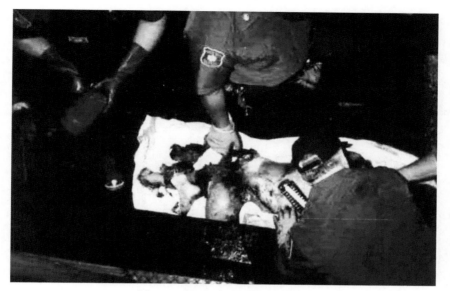

Man run over by subway train.

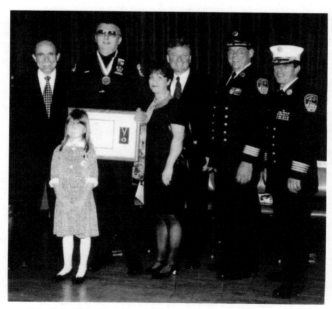

Medal of valor from Mayor Rudolph Giuliani

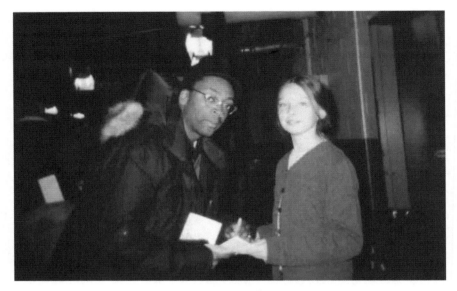

Hollie with Spike Lee

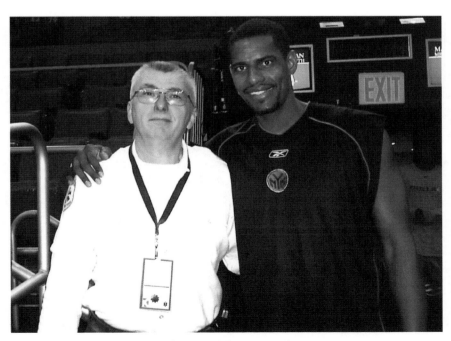

Knicks Kurt Thomas and me.

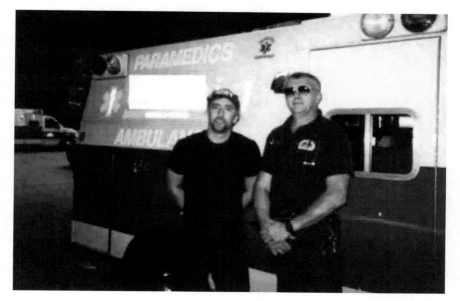

Nicolas Cage and me.

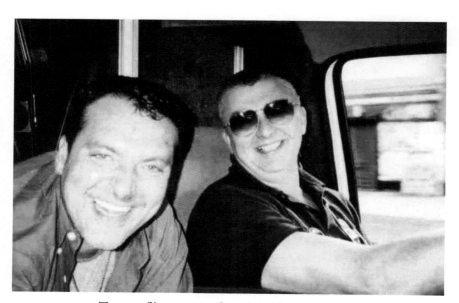

Tommy Sizemore and me laughing at the cabs.

BY NEW YORK CITY PARAMEDIC GEORGE STEFFENSEN

GEORGE'S BRAGGING PAGE

I'll try to impress you with what a great medic I am. O.K., I wasn't that great as a rookie. Come to think of it, I'm not even as good as I once was. I don't think that all the calls I did were perfect. I know I've taken a few trips up to see the medical director for some sort of protocol violation. Yikes I'm not a very good medic after all. I do have some awards and letters of commendation, so I've fooled some people.

Anyway, let me say this before the bragging begins. I stated in the introduction that most EMTs and medics go through their whole careers being great medics and EMTs without any recognition for their life-saving work. They have risked their lives to help people. No medals on their chests, no newspaper clippings. No plaques on their walls. Their families (I'm sure) are proud of them. However, just like the Cowardly Lion in the Wizard of Oz, it wasn't the medal that made him brave or the hero. These men and women of EMS do their jobs and do it well. They risk their lives and face many dangers. Don't believe for one second that because you can't see the hepatitis germs or the AIDS virus it can't kill you. You will be just as dead as from a bullet or the flames of a fire.

We too of the emergency medical services lost several paramedics and emergency medical technicians in the World Trade Center disaster. At shootings, fires, building collapses, any call where there are sick or injured, we are there. The men and women of the emergency medical services are the ones taking care of whoever needs medical attention. The people are not magically beamed over to the hospitals. They are treated and transported by highly trained paramedics and emergency medical technicians.

Over the years, I myself have been in some dangerous places and I know I wasn't alone. For example, under subway trains, in elevator shafts, in buildings which were on fire and buildings that were in danger of collapsing.

Unlike many of the men and women that I work hand in hand with, I have received lots of recognition for my work. I would like to thank those people who put me in for those awards. They do mean a lot to me, so I have to brag a bit. Well, really if you know me, I'll have to brag a lot. Someone once said if it's true it's not bragging, so I don't feel too guilty.

In my years with EMS, I have received over thirty pre-hospital save awards. This you get for successively resuscitating someone who, when you arrive on scene, has no pulse or respirations, basically dead. From Westchester County I received the Paramedic Of The Year Award for 1995. I was involved with two pediatric saves within a couple of months, along with a PBA life-saving award from New Castle police department in regards to one of the pediatric calls. I have also received several letters of commendation from the FDNY for my responses to major fires.

Last and my personal best is the Medal of Valor, which I received from Mayor Rudolph Giuliani and Thomas Von Essen, the Fire Commissioner of the City of New York.

This I received with my partner Andy for the rescue of the steel worker who fell while placing steel beams. He was up seven stories and we worked on him way up there. Then to get down to the ambulance the patient and I along with members of the police emergency service unit were brought down by a crane.

If you think seven stories isn't that high, look at the picture of my first jumper down. That was from six stories.

That is my bragging page. I hope you are impressed.

I just need to add (and want to brag for a second) about my father, who I didn't get to know for personal reasons. After he died I later found out that he was quite the war hero. He was in the Devil's Brigade, the first special forces of the Army. He received the Silver Star and Purple Heart along with others. I also have to brag about my brother who was with the 27th Marines in Vietnam; 1968 during the Tet offensive. He too has a chest full of ribbons. He has the Combat Action ribbon, Presidential Unit Citation and the Purple Heart, among others. I am very proud of them. They are true heroes.

So my EMS stuff doesn't impress anyone in my family. Hell, I can't even impress my wife. She too is a paramedic with the City of New York. She has her own commendations and stories to tell.

FIVE YEARS IN THE BIG CITY

No more rookie medic here. After over five years here in the city and the two years upstate before that, I can honestly say I know what I'm doing. I have been on lots of interesting calls. I have saved a number of people and have received several awards by now. I think I am one of the best medics around. Not a very modest one either. Yes, I'm pretty cocky; feeling good about what I have done.

The years on these tough streets have taught me not to be afraid of the homeless guys anymore. Going into Tompkins Square Park now means nothing to me. I am a seasoned medic and won't take crap from any drunk or junkie.

I have learned that I am the one in charge. I have been working out too. I want to ensure that when necessary I am ready and able to "help" someone if they need special "help."

I had never done weight training before and found that I was stronger now then when I was in the Marine Corps. I also did a lot on the Stairmaster machine. As a matter of fact, I did the 110 flights of the World Trade Center for a fundraiser. I did it in about 22 minutes.

I still like to buff jobs, but I can better judge now if the call is legitimate or not. If a call comes in for a shooting I listen first to see if more than one call has come in on it. If it is a real job several calls will come in for it. Unlike when I was a rookie, I thought if a call came in at all it must be real.

After racing to job after job to find the shooting is nothing at all, and the unconscious is the chronic drunk on the street, I have learned that it never comes in as what the dispatch center says. The buff belt has also lost a lot of equipment from it. No more big Mag-Lite. I always worked mostly day tours anyway. The fancy window punch no longer hanging from my belt. The pouch for my gloves is gone too. Enough gloves fit well in my back pocket. I no longer carry 14-gauge catheters in my shirt pocket for the trauma jobs. I still have the stethoscope around my neck. The oxygen wrench and trauma shears still together on my belt. Last, I still have the tourniquet on my belt.

I still get excited about the trauma jobs, the shootings, stabbings, the man under. (The man under refers to a person run over by a train.) The cardiac arrests, the saves; all-important to me and my big ego. Looking at my awards on the wall, my clippings from the newspapers. Calling home to set the VCR to catch myself on the news. I am pretty cool.

Well, at least I think so.

PARTNERS AND COWORKERS

Partners and co-workers are the people you work with. They sound the same but are far from the same, as I will explain. To me anyway, a co-worker is another paramedic that I work with who will be just as qualified as a medic. However, he or she will not be someone that I have grown to care about or one that I have been through anything important to move them into the small circle which I call partners.

A partner on the other hand is someone that you have been in some tough spots with and you know that they have your back as you have theirs. They have worked calls with you and you may have saved or lost a life together. Going into some dangerous situations, you feel confident when you are beside a partner, and nervous when just with a co-worker. When you are working with a partner the call flows smoothly, almost like synchronized swimming. You each know what the other is thinking and things get done automatically without a word spoken.

With a co-worker, the call turns into the Keystone Medics, you are both trying to do the same things and you are tripping over each other. You can't get on the same page so pretty much the patient care is compromised.

Partners look out for each other, even the small things that we do make a difference. Being sure to relieve your partner on time so he doesn't get caught with a late job all the time. Keeping the bus in good shape so he doesn't have to do double the work. Understanding if someone has a bad day and gets upset over something stupid. Knowing that they have lives at home and work isn't the only thing that could be upsetting them. Almost like being married.

Partners are a special group. Once they are in that circle you think of them as family. They may move away or change careers, but in our hearts we will always be close. Hey partners, I love you. Truly, the ones that I consider my partners, I really do love them. They have all touched me in some way and they will always be special to me.

9/11/2001

This date we know all too well. First, let's take a moment to remember all those rescue personnel who responded to their last and final call of duty. Their heroic efforts saved many, their sacrifices too great. Secondly we should take a moment to remember those people who were working there and gave their lives too. Many whose heroic efforts we will never know of.

September 11th, 2001 was a Tuesday and I was off that day. My wife, who is also a paramedic stationed in the Bronx was off as well. She was at our daughter's school. She liked helping out at school on her days off.

I was in bed resting when our son came running into our room to tell me what he had seen on the news bulletin: the World Trade Center had been hit by a plane. I couldn't believe what I was seeing and quickly was getting dressed as I continued to watch the news. I was just putting on my boots as I saw the tower collapse. This was so shocking; I didn't think that it would collapse. It had been struck at the upper floors. I had no idea that was even a possibility. It was definitely bad before the collapse but now I knew that the loss of firefighters, police and emergency medical workers was inevitable. Those numbers will be staggering. So many of them that I have worked with; the World Trade Center is in lower Manhattan where I've worked twelve years at this point.

I get in my car and head down to the disaster. I remind myself not to get too crazy; I have fifty miles to drive and getting into an accident will not get me there. My wife calls my cell phone and is very upset with me for going down there. "It is too dangerous, you don't know what else can happen," she screamed at me. She is right but I have to go. Later she too will find herself driving to the city as she is also called into work.

I drive down as far as Yonkers on Route 87, where the traffic is at a standstill. I need to get down there. I jump up onto the grass shoulder of the passing lane and try to get further. I have a Corvette, it is low to the ground. I am scraping at times but making my way. All of a sudden a van is behind me doing the same. I can't go any further as I can't get by the cars. I then realize that the van behind me is an unmarked police van from the city. Several cops jump out, one comes to my window, pissed at first and wondering what the hell am I doing. He sees my paramedic sticker in the window and tells me to follow their van when they get past the cars. Cops on foot start directing the other cars out of the way as we proceed past them. Ahead is a roadblock only allowing emergency personnel to pass. The van picks up speed as we head down towards the city. We pass a few more roadblocks, but with the police van in front we are moving pretty fast. By this time only emergency personal are in the convoy.

We get onto the FDR Drive, these cops in the van are doing eighty miles an hour and I'm right with them. I exit at 23rd Street to stop at my hospital to get equipment and to see what the best access is. There are a few of my partners there. They too have come in from their day off. There are no ambulances at our hospital to take. A police van is heading down to the disaster site. We ask for a ride down and the sergeant tells us to get in.

As we get near Ground Zero (as it will come to be called) it is very smoky and too quiet. By this time, the second tower has come down. I see one of our buses emerge from the smoke, heading out towards the hospital. One of our medics is driving but he is with someone who doesn't work with us. "Where is Andy?" I ask. He tells me they were with another patient when the second tower came down. It was so close to them that they were running for their lives. He was struck by a piece of debris, but fortunately he had his helmet on. He hasn't seen Andy after they were split up running from the falling tower. He couldn't say more, he needed to get his patient to the hospital.

After this there were lots of rescue personnel and ambulances waiting to get into the site but now there weren't patient to treat or transport. The devastation was beyond belief. Just trying to picture even where you were was difficult. The buildings, just rubble; you couldn't even get your bearings as to where you were.

Hours would pass and there wasn't anything for us to do but wait and hope. With no one to help we all felt so frustrated, wanting to do something. As night fell the area was lit by all kinds of emergency lights. You could hear the generators and the firefighters with their tools looking to find anyone possibly trapped, as well as their trucks pumping water to extinguish the many fires.

Later, one of our ambulances came by to bring us some food. Andy is back with his partner. He gets out and I give him a big hug. "Man I thought you got yourself killed when you were missing," I told him. Andy replied, "I thought I was going to die when we were running, when the second tower almost fell on us." "I'm glad to see you safe. I'll see you back at the hospital later," I told him. I felt so relieved that he was all right. Andy and I have worked Wednesdays together for several years and are very close. More time will pass with nothing to do. I never treated any patients that day. I felt so helpless and frustrated.

We are told to head back to our hospital. At this time it is 11 p.m. We need to talk with our supervisors and plan for the next day's assignments. The supervisor looks very distressed; she was involved from the beginning. We are outside together in the ambulance bay. Ground Zero is close by and we are still getting a lot of smoke as we stand there.

We are then informed that one of our emergency medical technicians is missing. Our hearts sink and I feel sick from the news. He was last seen going into the forward triage area in the lobby of the second tower just before it collapsed. We all knew what that meant but no one wanted to be the one who would give up hope.

This will be a great loss to all of us and of course so tragic for his young family. He is a young man with a great family; a wife and two small boys, their pictures proudly displayed in his locker.

David Marc Sullins, our EMT who heroically and tragically died on 9/11/2001.

So many firefighters, police and emergency medical personal died that awful day, as did so many innocent people. The weeks and months to come will be filled with funerals and services for so many young men and women: the firefighters, police, and emergency medical workers who gave the supreme sacrifice for strangers and friends.

You will never be forgotten.

THE PUDDLE

One early rainy morning, Andy Mazzola and I were dispatched to a cardiac call. The job was located at 345 East 47th Street. This was pretty far for us to go and the rain didn't help. We were driving up first Avenue as the rain poured down. The traffic was heavy and it was difficult to make any time. As we were getting near the United Nations building I was able to get into the bus lane. There weren't any buses at this point, and our ambulance was picking up speed. Things were getting a little better. I am keeping a close eye on the cars as I speed past them. All of a sudden Andy yells "George watch out!" I look but don't see any problem. "What?" I ask, as we are still moving pretty fast. "The puddle!" he yells.

Then out from the right side I see water like a tidal wave coming up from under our ambulance. Then out of the corner of my eye I notice a crowd at the bus station turning away. A whole group of people from the United Nations building all dressed in their expensive suits and dresses looking in horror as the wave of dirty street water comes crashing down on them. It looked like a giant wave from one of the surfing movies I've seen.

Andy said. "George did you see that?" but I could hardly see, I was laughing so hard. Then Andy started laughing too. I couldn't have gotten them any wetter if I had tried. We laughed the rest of the day every time we passed a bus stop.

To my surprise no one ever called to complain.

BY NEW YORK CITY PARAMEDIC GEORGE STEFFENSEN

ELEVATOR JOBS

MAN IN THE SHAFT

We were dispatched to an apartment building on Allen Street for a person in the elevator shaft. As we head down towards Allen Street, the police emergency service units are right in front of us. We follow them through the traffic and we are there in less than three minutes. As they get out of their trucks we get out of the ambulance and get our trauma gear. We enter the lobby of the building and the cops tell us that we need to go to the basement for the best access to the patient.

Once we are in the basement the cops are using a pry bar to force open the elevator doors. The doors slide open and expose the shaft. I can see the cables that raise and lower the elevator cars. I move closer and look down, seeing a male lying twisted at the bottom of the shaft, about six feet below where we are standing. The cop shines his flashlight down on the man. He looks badly injured, but I see his chest moving so I know he is breathing, at least. The cop yells down to him but gets no response. Definitely we need to work fast to get him to a trauma center. The emergency service sergeant tells us that until they secure the power, no one can enter the shaft.

It will take a few minutes for the cops to get to the roof to disable the power to the elevator. It seems longer when you are trying to rush. However the sergeant is right; scene safety takes precedence. Should the elevator come down while anyone is in the shaft it will just turn the rescuers into victims. I surely don't want to be crushed in there.

The power is turned off and we get the go ahead to go down to the patient. The cops go to get the Stokes basket and a ladder. I slide into the shaft, lowering myself down and then help my partner down with me. I know that the power is off but it still has me nervous. Something unexpected could happen and the elevator could come crashing down on us. We work fast and I keep one eye above me. If I even think something is wrong I'm getting out of here!

The patient is unconscious and has broken legs. We quickly intubate and immobilize him. The cops then slide a ladder down to us along with the Stokes basket. We place the patient on the long board and into the basket, then the cops tie ropes to the basket. As the cops pull the basket, sliding it up the ladder, my partner stays with the patient, as he needs to ventilate him. Once we are out we quickly get to our bus and get him to the local trauma center.

What had happened to him was that he was a deliveryman with some boxes and had his back to the elevator doors. He was waiting on the third floor. The elevator malfunctioned and its doors opened but the car wasn't there. The deliveryman never looked and just backed into the elevator with the dolly. Before he knew it, it was too late and he fell the four stories.

He did arrive at the emergency room with a good pulse and blood pressure, but I don't know what happened after that.

DIFFICULTY BREATHING IN ELEVATOR

The difficulty breather in the stuck, occupied elevator is a job we get often. Every time an elevator gets stuck in a building the 911 call comes in. No one will ever say they are just stuck in the elevator. They always have to add that someone has trouble breathing. This is sure to get a faster response (along with the Fire Department) because of course if you have trouble you definitely need an ambulance.

So job after job, the difficulty breather in the stuck occupied elevator will come in. Sure enough, the Fire Department comes and the ambulance crews are there, waiting to help these people. The doors will be pried open and all the people will exit the elevator and be just fine.

Yes, I'm happy that everyone is fine. I just wish they wouldn't say that they have trouble breathing to get a faster response. Everyone only thinks of themselves. They never give it a second thought that by telling the 911 dispatcher that a person has trouble might delay a person who is truly having difficulty breathing.

I never take the time to try to educate them, as I know my words will fall on deaf ears.

BY NEW YORK CITY PARAMEDIC GEORGE STEFFENSEN

FIRE CALLS

FIREFIGHTER DOWN

One afternoon I was working with a young paramedic. We are good friends and, as a matter of fact, went on a cruise together: my wife and I, and Hamlet and his future bride. We had a great time together. I took him scuba diving for his first time. The girls hung out on the beach. At night the dinners on the ship were amazing. Hamlet came to our department as an emergency medical technician and had finished paramedic training about a year ago by this time. Later on, he will advance past me and become my boss. I'm proud of him; he is a great boss and a true partner.

We were just completing a call and were pulling out of Bellevue's emergency room. Across the FDR Drive we could see smoke coming from a thirty-story apartment building. We can hear the fire trucks responding but there are no fire trucks on the scene yet. I heard a window break and now thick, heavy smoke is pouring out from several windows. Where the smoke is coming from is up at about the nineteenth floor.

We are just across the drive and can get there pretty fast. Hamlet looks at me as if to say should we buff this? I smiled at my young friend and say, "Go ahead. Let's get on it."

This looks like it is going to be a big job. I like doing calls that are out of the ordinary anyway. We called to the dispatcher, advised them of the fire and requested to be put on the job. To our surprise, the dispatcher said it isn't coming in as a major alarm and a basic unit is in route. We were both a bit annoyed. I guess from the dispatch center the dispatcher must have a better view of things than we do. Well, we are not disappointed for long. We have only gone one block when the dispatcher is sending us to the fire after all.

The fire has been upgraded to a second alarm. My foot goes to the floor, as I know other units might try to get there first and cancel us. This is right in our area and we won't let that happen.

We pull up in front of the building and a fire captain directs us to where he wants us to station our bus. Before we are parked he comes running to us and tells us a fireman is down on the twentieth floor, a mayday call as he put it. This is very unusual for them to ask us to go to the fire floor, so we know that this means the firefighter is either unconscious or in cardiac arrest.

We have all of our equipment: the drug bag (which also has the intubation equipment), the cardiac monitor, oxygen, and a long board. We have to climb up two flights of stairs outside the building just to get to the lobby. Our hearts are already racing, partly from the adrenalin and partly from the physical strain of carrying this stuff up the two flights. Time is an enemy to someone who is in need of oxygen or CPR.

First I'm afraid of what might be wrong with this firefighter, knowing full well that it will be a firefighter that we work with on a daily basis. Secondly, we are running into this fire with just helmets on our heads and our medical equipment in hand. We don't have the air tanks or special bunker gear the firefighters have on.

We are at the lobby and are told there is a firefighter down on the twentieth floor. The electricity is out there are no elevators to take us up. Thank God for adrenalin as we head into the poorly lit stairwell. The first few stories aren't too bad as we are rushing past other firefighters who are heading up the stairs to fight the fire. We recognize most of them as we move past them. I fear for their safety too, this job already has one firefighter down.

I'm up to the tenth floor now and the stairwell is smoky. I am coughing from the smoke. Water is running down the steps like a waterfall, making them slippery as ice as we struggle to get to the firefighter. At first I am bothered by the water getting me wet and the stairs being so dangerous. This is just adding to a bad situation. I look back to my partner and notice he is lagging behind a bit. I yell down to him, "Hammy, are you okay?" He yells back, "I'm right behind you, go ahead, I'll be good." Knowing that he is okay and that the firemen in the stairwell are close to him, I push myself harder up the stairs. I try my best to get up those stairs, through the smoke that has gotten much thicker now. By this time I am soaked and dirty from the water pouring down the stairs and the soot from the fire. I'm short of breath, my heart racing even faster than before.

I have made it to the eighteen floor. Two more flights, I can make it,

I'm telling myself. Forget about your bad knees; forget your heart racing in your chest. Knowing that the firefighter is depending on us. Finally I push open the stairwell doors to the twentieth floor.

Some firefighters are in there and they yell to me that the guy is on the twenty-second floor. Back up the stairs I go and again push open the doors this time to the twenty-second floor.

One fireman is sitting up against the wall, sweat pouring off of him. His color is pale but he is conscious and alert. I ask where is the firefighter you called EMS for and they say it is for him. I ask again "are you sure?" and they are definite. Good, I just want to be sure. In the confusion I don't want to be helping a minor problem if there is a guy unconscious or in cardiac arrest in a different room.

I am very relieved that he is doing better. He had passed out from too much smoke and heat. Now he just needs some oxygen and rest and he will be fine. The two things I'm carrying are the monitor and the drug bag. My young partner has the oxygen and long board. He is not up to the twenty-second floor yet. I head back down the stairs to meet him to get the oxygen.

Hell, he is down five flights before I meet him. I advise him the firefighter is good, he just needs some oxygen and rest. I grab the oxygen bag and rush back to the firefighter. After a little bit my exhausted partner is working on another firefighter who has a laceration to his hand. I look over when I notice that the long board is not in sight. I say, "Hey Hammy, where is the long board?" He answers, "Hell, I got rid of that on the third floor!" I just laugh and shake my head.

Things are looking better by this time. We are treating some minor injuries, giving some oxygen to firefighters who have taken in too much smoke. The fire is getting under control. Fortunately no one was badly injured.

That was quite a scare we had when we were heading up those stairs. It could have been a lot worse. Finally we are advised by our EMS captain that we are relieved and may head down to our bus.

Going down these stairs is a lot easier then going up with all the equipment. Knowing that everyone is doing well is a great feeling. While resting at the back of our ambulance a Fire Chief comes over to us. "Guys, I want to thank you for your work up there. Several of the men wanted me to let you

BY NEW YORK CITY PARAMEDIC GEORGE STEFFENSEN

know that you guys did a good job for us. Thanks again."

We looked like messes, both soaked with our faces black from the soot. This was a cool job. Even better, this will be the last job of this shift. "Central, show this unit going back to the hospital, restock and tour change."

I tease Hamlet a bit as we head back to the hospital. "You left the long board on the third floor? I had to come back for the oxygen. You better start doing the stair master machine on your days off like I do. I'm forty seven and you are twenty one, you should carry *me* up the stairs!"

SEVENTEENTH STREET JOB

It's the start of our shift; just a little past seven in the morning and we're having our coffee as we sit in the bus. We are sitting at 20th Street and 3rd Avenue when our unit is dispatched to a major burn call. The call is on 17th Street and 3rd Avenue; we are only three blocks away. Burn calls are not that frequent (at least for me) and I'm not so comfortable doing them. As we pull onto the scene we are in front of a restaurant. We get our stretcher and the rest of our equipment and move towards the restaurant. My partner is pulling the stretcher and I'm behind it as we get to the front door. I stop when I see in front of me a man who is smoldering; his clothes are burnt off him. I stop the stretcher as my partner tells me to go inside. I say, "I think the call is for this guy!" He looks at the smoldering guy.

We quickly get him onto the stretcher and pour sterile water on him to stop the burning. He is burnt very badly; the only clothes left on him are his work boots. He has parts of a shirt and pants which are almost burnt completely off. I can't believe what I see. This is one of the worst burns I've ever seen and this man is standing and able to walk and talk. I can't even tell what race this guy is; his face and hair are so severely burned. The burns are so deep that they aren't painful. There isn't too much that we need to do for him. Getting him to a specialty burn hospital is the best we can do. We wrap him in burn sheets; we had already stopped the burning process when we poured the sterile water on him. His airway is good. We give him oxygen and check his lungs sounds; they are good too. He doesn't need any morphine as he doesn't have much pain. I call the dispatcher to have the specialty burn hospital to be on standby for this patient.

What had happened to this young man was that he was working on a garbage truck. When he threw a can of garbage into the back of the truck, it exploded into a massive ball of fire. It is very hard looking at him as we raced to the hospital. I look for a vein to place an IV so I can give him some fluids on the way. I find one small place that hasn't been too burned and put the IV in. While talking to him on the way I find out he is twenty-four, just married. How sad is this, having this young newlywed so burnt and knowing that no matter what, his injuries will surely kill him within the next few days.

Later I tell my partner, "I guess your coffee hadn't kicked in yet. I can't believe you walked right past that poor guy smoldering and didn't realize that he was the patient."

SLICE

I don't want to leave this funny story out. Slice is one of my partners. He truly is a great paramedic. At times he is a bit intense but definitely a medic you want working on you. He doesn't let many people get close to him. I try my best to be a good partner to him.

I don't know what it is like to be a black man, so I can't understand the times when he thinks someone is looking to get him in trouble because he is black. I know that there are people out there that are like that so I know that his thoughts are not always unjustified. Sad to say, but for this story you need to have a little understanding of my partner Slice.

Slice is a guy who comes to work and is very serious about being a paramedic. He gets upset when the other medics are lazy and don't do the right things. He feels that everyone should pull his or her weight. He is absolutely correct and I agree when he gets upset at his "partners" for not doing what they should.

He is a pretty tough guy and most people don't want to get on his bad side. He is honest with the other medics. If you are not a good paramedic he has no problem letting you know. I know that when you have an incompetent medic working with you it makes all medics look bad.

I have to say it made me feel good when Slice told me that if he went down, I was one of the few he would let work on him.

So let's get to the funny call, which came in at 10:15 p.m. for a difficulty breathing. Another late job and we are on the back end of a double shift. Late jobs are bad enough, but after 15 hours you really don't want a late call.

We go inside a church where the patient is found sitting in a chair. She seems to be a little confused as we rapidly place her on the stretcher. A quick assessment shows that her vital signs are stable. The trouble breathing comes from her walking too far with her history of emphysema. She also has a history of Alzheimer's.

I place her on some oxygen and her breathing trouble is resolved. Due to her age (and also to be on the safe side) we prepare to take her to the hospital.

Slice starts to question her to get the information for the ambulance call report now that her condition has been treated.

First he gets her name from her. Then he asks her age and again the patient answers him. Slice is asking the questions quickly to try to get this over with so we can get out on time.

Then he asks the question, "Where do you live?" The patient looks at Slice and doesn't answer. Slice asks again, "Where do you live?" and this time I hear frustration in his voice. The old lady looks a little nervous under the oxygen mask. Then Slice says, (as he shows her the paperwork) "Look lady, you don't have anything I want. I'm not going to come rob you, I need it for the report!"

I almost fell out of the ambulance laughing. Then I said to Slice, "I know you are stressed about this late job, I guess you forgot she has Alzheimer's." Slice looked at the old lady and gently patted her on the head and told her, "Don't worry, we'll get it later."

He ended the questions and we headed to the hospital. The nurses with security can go through her purse and get more information later.

We got her to the hospital and when we pulled into the ambulance bay a family member was waiting for their grandmother. Everything worked out well. She was fine and we got off on time.

THE ARREST ON THE BOWERY

One evening we were dispatched to 208, The Bowery. This location was one we would be sent to numerous times. We would get sent there for the shooting, the cop shot, the cardiac arrest. Lots of calls at this location are unfounded. After the third time being sent to this location for apparently no reason, a cop told me that it was a Chinese whorehouse and its competitor would call these jobs in to disrupt business.

This night would be very different. Usually, when we knocked on the door for access it would take literally five minutes for them to let us in. By that time they were able to get things looking more legitimate before we could get upstairs. Instead the doors flew open and a small Chinese man lead us up the stairs to a room.

We entered the room with all our medic equipment for the cardiac arrest. There, naked in the middle of the floor, was a girl who looked about twelve years old. I immediately checked for a pulse or breathing. She was not breathing and had no pulse! I started CPR and my partner called for backup, confirming the arrest. He then quickly placed the paddles on her chest to check her rhythm. She was flat line, asystole. My partner took over compressions and I place the breathing tube. By this time the basic unit was on scene they took over ventilations and compressions as my partner got the intravenous line established. Once the line was in placed he pushed one milligram of epinephrine and then one milligram of atropine.

We stop CPR for a moment to check the patient and the monitor. Damn, no change; we repeat the medications and continue CPR. After a minute or two we stop again to check, still no change. Let's try some Narcan and some dextrose. The medications again are given. More CPR, another round of epi and atropine. A few more minutes pass still no change. Still a flat line, not even something worth shocking. It looks very bad for this little girl. We continue CPR for a few more minutes, giving epi now about every 4 minutes.

We haven't seen a sign of hope; and we certainly have taken appropriate action. Last thing to do is call the telemetry doctor to get permission to terminate. I call the doctor and give my report while the crew continues to work her up in the event the doctor wants us to try anything else or wants us to transport her.

The doctor says, "It sounds like you did the right things. Nothing on the monitor after all the medications, correct?" "Yes, we checked in three leads and nothing!" I reply. "Just because of her age, let's just try an amp of bicarb and defibrillate her at 200 joules," he says. "Then if you still have asystole you can call it."

It can only help, but we all think this is going to be a fruitless effort. We have been around and asystole for over twenty minutes with all the stuff she has received doesn't improve. My partner pushes the bicarb, we do CPR for a minute to push it around a bit and then I charge the paddles. Paddles charge to 200 joules as I call clear, check to make sure no one is touching her, and then defibrillate.

Her small body jumps from the current going into her. Then we look to see if anything happened. I can't believe what I see on the monitor: a beautiful, tight complex sinus rhythm with a rate of 130 beats per minute. We all know (or let me say, paramedics know) that you can have a nice-looking rhythm on the monitor without a pulse. Quickly I look at her neck and I see a bounding pulse. This is truly short of a miracle, and if I weren't there I wouldn't believe it myself. We check her blood pressure and it's 110/64; fantastic!

Next we bolus her with lidocaine and then get her ready to transport her to the emergency room. Then down to the ambulance. We monitor her vital signs as we rush her to our emergency room. I call ahead and tell the doctor the amazing news. They are waiting as we pull up to the hospital.

Her vital signs remain stable and she gets admitted to the cardiac care unit. Even more crazy unbelievable stuff. After one week in the hospital this young girl who happened to be twenty years old will be discharged without any deficits. This was really an amazing job. As a footnote, 208 The Bowery is no longer a whorehouse. So save yourself the trip.

A QUICK FUNNY ARREST

We arrived at an apartment for a chest pain when a ninety-plus woman answered the door. As soon as we stepped in, she collapsed and went into cardiac arrest. Hell the lady is ninety plus; I feel bad starting on her. She is easily intubated and an intravenous is started. The monitor shows asystole, so she gets the epi and atropine. We go though the proper steps waiting to see any change, so far nothing.

At this time the police come into the apartment as I'm calling the doctor to get orders to pronounce her. The sergeant asks if we are going to take her. Sorry, but we are on the phone and are getting orders to terminate.

The cops don't like us leaving the bodies as it ties them up by staying with them until the medical examiner comes. We get the orders to terminate and my partner does the paper work. As I'm bullshitting with the sergeant, I haven't yet removed the cables from the "dead" lady. All of a sudden the sergeant smiles and tells me, "Hey, there are bumps on the monitor!" I look over and sure enough there are "bumps" on the monitor.

Now what? Okay, let's check for a pulse. Sure enough, she has one of those too. Lucky for us I was lazy and all the stuff had not yet been removed. With the breathing tube in place and the IV still in we just needed to place her on our stretcher and keep an eye on her vital signs.

This made the sergeant very happy. He even said that, after seeing us revive this ninety-year-old lady by hardly trying, "if I go into arrest or get shot I want you guys!" We laughed as we left the scene. The lady will die in the emergency room. All those drugs just gave her a few more minutes. It was her time.

JUST FOR THE RECORD

I only did these two arrest stories. As I looked at them I realized that it was two calls I was ready to give up on, one that had an amazing ending. Those two were just weird ones. You would be bored to death to read job after job of the cardiac arrest saves! Again, just for the record, remember over thirty pre hospital saves. How many confirmed kills? That we will never know!

BY NEW YORK CITY PARAMEDIC GEORGE STEFFENSEN

HONEY DON'T LOOK IN THE BEDROOM

It was about 2:00 p.m. when we were assigned to the cardiac arrest in an apartment. When we entered the apartment the lady who opened the door quickly pointed to the bedroom. There we found a man about fifty years old in cardiac arrest. My partner and I moved him to the floor and proceeded to work on him. He was flat line and we tried everything we could, but there was no change.

We called our telemetry doctor and give report and requested to terminate, which means to stop our resuscitative efforts. The doctor gave us permission to terminate. We stop our resuscitate efforts and record the time of death.

At this time the police have arrived on scene, and I went to give my condolences to the wife. I went into the living room, giving her the same speech that I have done lots of times. "Sorry, we did everything we could but he died." Before I could get his information from her she frantically screamed, "You have to take him!"

I explained to her that we had already done everything we could and with the authorization from the telemetry physician, we would be leaving. The police would be there until someone from the medical examiner's office arrived.

She became very upset and said, "No, you must take him. You don't understand! You must take him before my husband gets home."

Well, now that is a big problem. As much as I would have liked to help her, we had already pronounced his death. We had already given the police the time of death. Plus with any untimely death, this is a case for the medical examiner's office.

The bedroom will be considered a crime scene until it is determined that his death was from natural causes. This would have been the case even if it had been her husband. However, this not being her husband, and having a naked dead man in her bed will likely raise some questions.

I sure don't want to be there when her husband gets home. This is not something that he is going to find as amusing as I do. To find his bed is roped off with crime scene tape should make for some interesting conversation at dinner. "Hi honey, don't go in the bedroom. There is a naked dead guy in there, please pass the gravy."

One thing I always say about our job: when I see other people's problems, my problems seem so small.

FAMOUS PEOPLE

I have had the opportunity to meet several famous people during the course of my paramedic career. I have done some standbys for some movie shoots. I also work with an ambulance service that has the contracts with Madison Square Garden and Yankee Stadium, as well as other high profile sports and entertainment facilities.

When Nicolas Cage and Tom Sizemore were looking to ride with New York City paramedics while researching their roles for the movie Bringing Out The Dead, I was the lucky one that took them both out on calls with me. Just for the record, they treated us all great. It was fun doing calls with them. They both took pictures with us and gave us autographs. Tommy Sizemore gave me an autograph for my kids that said, "Your dad is a true American hero," signed, Tom Sizemore. I thought that was really nice for my kids.

Nicolas Cage rode one night and Tommy Sizemore another. When they would enter the apartments, the people would start talking to them and forget about why they called an ambulance.

Nicolas Cage took the roll of the observer, watching what we were doing as we would access the patients. Tommy Sizemore was a bit more involved. He had us all laughing, as he would curse out of the window at taxicabs that didn't get out of our way fast enough. I had to tell my boss that if any complaints came in when Tommy Sizemore was riding, it was his fault.

While working at Madison Square Garden I get to meet famous people there too. The players, the famous guests like Spike Lee, the different performers at the concerts. What a great job, to get paid to go to these great events. Our daughter Hollie has been to a number of games and was happy to meet these people. She has some pictures and autographs from players and other famous people.

BY NEW YORK CITY PARAMEDIC GEORGE STEFFENSEN

ON THE JOB INJURIES

On the job injuries are very common doing our job. Besides the dangers of driving in adverse conditions, we face people who are mentally unstable, as well as a number of people under the influence of drugs and alcohol. Anytime you enter a building, there is potential danger. Unaware of a drug deal going on as you enter a poorly lit stairwell, wearing a uniform and carrying a radio; being mistaken for the police is not unusual.

Putting that aside, the job is very physical. Carrying people who are very heavy and having to lift them from awkward positions is very difficult and back injuries are common.

To give you an idea of how common injuries on the job are, my family alone is a great example. I myself have had two operations to repair injuries I sustained on the job. My wife Luci, a paramedic in the Bronx, injured her neck and back and needs surgery to repair those injuries; they are very bad. She most likely will not be able to return working as a paramedic again. Our daughter Jennifer is an emergency medical technician intermediate out in Ohio. She too has been injured. She was in an accident where her ambulance flipped. She had to undergo surgery as well.

So three out of three people in my family working in EMS has had serious injuries that required surgery. It looks like my wife Luci wins the prize for most serious. I feel very bad seeing her in pain. I hope after her surgery and rehabilitation she will feel much better.

I'm a pretty big man. I don't know how these smaller men and women are able to do this job. I know that I struggle on a number of calls. I'm amazed that they are able to do the job.

BY NEW YORK CITY PARAMEDIC GEORGE STEFFENSEN

SUBWAY JOBS

The subway system is very large and a bit confusing. It is a whole different way of life in the subway. The people are different; they are always in some sort of a rush. Everyone seems to not look at each other, so as not to offend someone. You are always aware of the dangers down here. Am I going to get mugged, shot, or maybe pushed onto the track in front of a train as it comes speeding into the station? These things enter my mind when I go in there. I don't ride the subways very often but when I do, I am very aware of my surroundings.

Doing calls in the subway is difficult in many ways. One problem is that when you are down there, your radio is useless. Being able to reach the dispatcher is your lifeline when things go wrong. So down there in the subways we are on our own; we won't be able to get help should we run into a problem. We also can't get more information should we need directions to locate the patient. Another problem we face is that the system is so big, the callers don't always know the exact location. We find ourselves walking the uptown platforms and then the downtown platforms before we can locate the patient. We lose valuable time on those jobs where seconds count. We also have to walk great distances from the ambulance to reach the patients. It becomes routine to bring all of your medic equipment down with you as it would take too long to retrieve it should the patient's condition not match the call type. This is especially true if you are working with my partner Andy E. who we call Carry All. He requires you to bring all the equipment on every call no matter how close, and no matter how minor.

Some calls, when you are close enough to the ambulance and if the call comes in for trouble breathing, you might just bring the stair chair and oxygen. In the event the patient is unconscious you can quickly retrieve the drug bag and monitor. This would not work down in the subway, as it would take several minutes to run back to the ambulance. Then several more minutes to get back to the patient.

Finally, the last common problem we face as we try to make our way to the patient is that everyone else is more important than the patient. People will push us out of the way so they won't miss their train. As I said at the beginning they don't even look up to notice that you are in uniform carrying all this heavy medical equipment. Most of them wouldn't care unless it is for them or a loved one anyway. Then of course the guy the day before who wouldn't let you down the stairs will be the same guy complaining, "What took you so long to get here?"

MAN UNDER

The man under call is a job that refers to a person who has fallen or jumped onto the tracks of a subway train. Friday night at about 5:00 p.m. we are dispatched to a man under at the 14th Street Union Square Station on the northbound L line. We are there in a couple of minutes. I grab the long board and oxygen bag. My partner grabs the trauma bag and c-collar. Then we make our way through the sea of people exiting the station. I feel like a salmon going upstream, as I have to push my way past all these people. Rush hour is bad timing for a subway job no matter what the call. When seconds count, it is really bad. After making our way to the platform I can see some Transit Police are there, and they have spotted the man. He is near the end of the platform under the train. The train is so huge and heavy it is really scary for me. I hate going under cars and going under a train is much worse. I go between the two subway cars closest to the patient. I squeeze myself in the opening between the train and the platform, all the time worrying if the train should move a bit while I'm doing this I will be crushed. I get under the train now and see a flashlight from one of the transit cops who is with the patient. Nervously I make my way to them. Still worried if the train moves and the other danger of being electrocuted should I accidentally touch the third rail which powers this massive machine. The track bed is very dirty and has puddles of water that make this situation unpleasant on top of the dangers.

I get my first look at the patient. Seeing his body with his arms and legs in unnatural positions I know he is in very bad shape, if he isn't already dead. I hear him moan as I get a little closer. Well, he isn't dead, that's something good. There is blood coming from his right upper arm and blood coming from his left thigh. Both of these extremities are in positions they normally can't be in, so I'm sure he has open fractures at least. He has a heavy jacket and blue jeans on so we will have to get them out of the way to see what is going on and treat his injuries. As with any patient, especially with extensive trauma patients, it is important to get to the basics first, and then go with your head to toe inspection.

All right then, lets get to the basics. My partner has been right with me; he loves being under trains as much as I do. He stabilizes the patient's head and neck as we check his airway and breathing, the first things we need to do. He places the c-collar to prevent him from moving his head and neck as we see he has injuries to his head. He also puts him on oxygen, another thing that is done automatically. Oxygen is routinely given to anyone who has sustained major injuries.

Okay, his airway and breathing are good and he has a decent radial pulse. We need to see what his injuries are and control his bleeding. Certainly we are aware of the right arm and left leg, but we must check further to ensure we don't miss something else by just treating the obvious. With the help of the transit cops we carefully roll the patient onto his side and place the long board next to him. I quickly cut open the back of this coat and shirt and inspect his back. His back is bruised but no cuts to his back, his ribs feel even with no obvious fractures and he has equal lung expansion; this is all good. I cut the back of his pants to check the rest of his back area before we roll him onto the long board. Then I cut the rest of his jacket and shirt off. His chest is fine, but as I remove the jacket and shirt I see that his right arm is not an open fracture as I had thought. His arm has been nearly severed off at the shoulder and is only hanging on by some skin and muscle.

One of the cops takes over holding stabilization of the head and neck as my partner grabs a trauma dressing and wraps the shoulder and places it into a more natural position. Fortunately for us the patient is pretty out of it from head trauma so we don't need to worry about sedation for him. The left arm is fine and we will use it for the IVs and to check his blood pressure. Moving further down, his abdomen is soft and looks normal on gross inspection. I cut his pants off now and his left leg has also been nearly severed as well. It too is hanging on only by some small pieces of skin and muscle. His right leg is fine; nothing obvious there. My partner takes another trauma dressing and wraps the left thigh, stopping the bleeding there as well.

My partner gets a trauma line set up while I secure him to the long board. By the time I have secured the patient to the long board and the transit cops are ready to help carry him, my partner has established the intravenous line. With someone on each corner, we carry the patient out of the subway and into our bus.

A good thing about a job like this is that with all the transit cops with us, carrying is a lot easier. Plus they clear the people out of the way so we are not impeded at all. Once we are in the ambulance, I give a notification to the hospital and the trauma team is waiting for us.

The injuries are very severe; he will lose his leg and his right arm, but he will make it.

I never found out what happened or how he ended up under the train in the first place.

BY NEW YORK CITY PARAMEDIC GEORGE STEFFENSEN

COCAINE OVERDOSE

One afternoon, I was working with my partner Andy E. when we are dispatched to the corner of Avenue C and East Houston for an unconscious male about twenty-five-years-old. As soon as we get on scene and see the patient, right away he looks in bad shape. Just looking at him we see that his color is extremely pale and sweat is just pouring off him. We quickly get him on the stretcher and into our bus so we can work on him. I call for a basic unit to back us up. He looks like he could code at any second. The patient is very out of it so Andy checks his airway and tries to put in an oral airway in. I check for a radial pulse on his left arm, no distal pulse: he is in shock. I quickly put the monitor on him to check his heart rate. Wow, his rate is over 230 beats per minute. Judging by his condition and seeing the track marks it would be a good guess to think he was shooting cocaine.

Although he only responds to painful stimuli, he still has a gag reflex. Andy removes the oral airway and places him on 100 percent oxygen. I check for a vein on the right arm. Nothing, and I mean nothing there. Andy checks his left arm and sees the track marks and some abscesses but no veins for him to try for. Fortunately he does have a great external jugular vein. I place a 16-gauge large bore catheter there with a 1000cc bag of fluid to try to bring up his pressure.

At this time the basic unit is there to give us a hand. We have him on oxygen and a line is in place. He could use a second one, but one is good enough as he has such poor access. He is still in shock, and I tell Andy I think we should try to cardiovert him, which basically means to shock him. Andy doesn't think it will help because his rate is cocaine-induced. I know what you are thinking but it might help.

Like the show, Who Wants To Be A Millionaire, let's phone a friend and see what they suggest. Not exactly; what I mean is that when two medics don't agree, you can call the telemetry doctor and get their advice. I call the doctor and he thinks it is worth it to try the one-shock cardiovert once and then transport.

Andy doesn't like it; he's driving and goes up to the front. I'm in the back with one of the EMTs getting ready to blast this guy. I call up to Andy and tell him if he goes into arrest after I shock him please, come back and give me a hand.

There is no need to sedate the patient, he is pretty out of it and the sedation could lower his blood pressure more. Let's do this. I charge the paddles to 100 joules, hit the sync button and say clear. I check to make sure no one is touching the patient. Then I shock him.

"Aahhh!" the patient screams, almost giving me a heart attack. Then he lies quiet again. I check the monitor; no change. I call up to Andy, "Hey Andy, you were right, no change. Could you please race us to the hospital now?"

We let the emergency room know we will be there in about four minutes and advise them of the patient's condition.

We bring the patient into one of the slots and the rookie doctor comes in. He sees the monitor and sees we only have the one external jugular line. He gets some catheters and looks at the left arm in an effort to place a second line. He looks but just like we said, there is nothing really to try for there. The patient used up all those veins up shooting heroin and coke.

He asks me, "What do you have over there?" as he continues looking at the left arm. I tell him, "Absolutely nothing!" He says in a very arrogant way, "Let me look!" and he brings the catheters over to the right side of the bed, ready to show me that he will get the line.

To his surprise I am right, there is nothing there, not even an arm. It had been amputated years ago, most likely from an infection from shooting drugs. No arm at all from the shoulder down. I look at the rookie doctor and say, "The next time when I say nothing, you will believe me!"

THE DRUNK GIRL

Here we go, dispatched to the unconscious at East 19th Street and 1st Avenue. The job is very close to where we are sitting and we pull on scene in a minute. This location is one that is way too familiar to us. This is where one of our regular drunk guys hangs out. So we know who we expect to find.

Well ladies and gentlemen, we are wrong; well, semi-wrong. It is a drunk, but not our regular guy. This drunk is a young girl about twenty-years-old, very pretty and very drunk. She is with a young man who is sober, and he is the one who called the ambulance. He tells us that she was out from the hospital's alcohol rehab unit and obviously drank while out on her pass. He quickly leaves the scene before we can get more information from him.

We pour her onto the stretcher, as she is as limp as a wet noodle. We start to check her vital signs and try to get some basic information from her. She looks at us and asks, "What are we doing?" We explain (as best as you can explain to a drunk) that we are here helping you and that we're going to take you back to the hospital. To this she replies, "You know what I need." I'm thinking, not another drink. She says, "I need a big cock in me." I'm shocked and say, "Well, that leaves me out." Wow, I sure would not have picked that as a possible answer.

Let me tell you something, although this sounds like a funny call, later it can be funny, but right now I'm shitting pickles. No one with half a brain wants a drunk girl talking like this in their bus.. This could be big trouble down the road. So we treat her like a major trauma. We want her out of our bus as fast as possible. Let me explain how fast I want her out of our bus: I drive down 1st Avenue the wrong way several blocks to get her to the emergency room.

The dispatcher keeps track of the time you arrive on scene, the time you spent on scene, and then your time from scene to the hospital. I know my time from scene to the emergency room has to be some sort of record. Once we arrived in the emergency room things don't get much better. She continues to say things that were way inappropriate. I think I turned several shades of red while waiting for the triage nurse.

The sad thing is that this poor girl really does have a big problem. Hopefully she will get back to the rehab unit and get back to a better way of life.

FLOATERS

We get dispatched to a number of calls where a person is in the river, be it the Hudson River on the west side or the East River, which is more in my area.

One morning I had a woman who had jumped into the East River in the middle of December to rescue her puppy who had fallen in. She was in good shape and was able to get to the puppy. When she reached him she was too cold and unable to get back to shore. Lucky for her, some other bystanders were able to reach her with some long boards and helped her and the puppy get back on shore.

We arrived to find her extremely hypothermic as well as the puppy too. We took her and her puppy to the hospital. They placed her in the emergency room with special warming blankets. We put the cute little puppy in our locker room and put warm blankets on him too. They both did well and were safely home by the end of the night.

Not everyone who is taken from the East River is as lucky as she was. On more then a few occasions we have seen people pulled from the river who had been in there for weeks. I recall one hot summer we were sent down for a man in the water near the South Street Seaport. There were several police emergency trucks with their divers, along with some police harbor boats.

It was about 6:30 at night and a big crowd was gathering to see what was going on. One of the harbor units was able to grab hold of the body and was pulling it to the pier to bring it up on land. It was obviously a dead man, and he was very badly decomposed. This we heard over the police radio. As the harbor boat came into the pier the crowd was really big. When they were able to lift him out of the water and place him on the ground everyone could see and smell this horrible sight.

The crowd was gone in seconds. I hope it didn't spoil their dinner plans.

BY NEW YORK CITY PARAMEDIC GEORGE STEFFENSEN

HOMICIDE

The first homicide that I remember was a call that we were dispatched to on Water Street. Over the police radio we hear several police units being dispatched to a domestic dispute at 222 Water Street, apartment 23. The police dispatcher advises the units that numerous calls are coming in on it. Jobs that have many calls coming in on them turn out to be very serious. As we listen to the radio to hear the units getting on scene we start heading towards the call in case an ambulance is needed. Sure enough once the police are on the scene they are requesting a bus forthwith.

"Central, rush the bus. We have a woman in cardiac arrest!" the cop calls over his radio.

My partner and I head down the FDR Drive as we tell our dispatcher we will be on scene in two minutes. We pull on scene in the two minutes and get our stretcher and equipment and head up to the apartment. The ride up to the 20th floor in the elevator seems like a lifetime.

As the doors to the elevator open we see cops wrestling with a man. They subdue him and handcuff him. To our left other cops are in the hall doing CPR on a bloody woman who looks about forty. Around the woman there is a lot of blood and what looks like broken wine bottles. My partner and I join the cops and start working on the woman. My partner takes care of the airway and I get the trauma lines in place.

I can see into the apartment where the woman had been. There are broken wine bottles, turned over chairs, blood and wine mixed together in big pools. Looking at the apartment and seeing her injuries, she had put up some fight. I can see the defense wounds to her hands where she has deep lacerations exposing some tendons. There is hair mixed into these lacerations. I assume they are from the man she desperately tried to fight off.

It upsets me to think that with all these people in the building hearing her screams and calling 911 that no one would try to help this poor woman. They will have to live with her death.

BY NEW YORK CITY PARAMEDIC GEORGE STEFFENSEN

Although we got her to the hospital in less than ten minutes with the advance life support procedures, she did not survive this brutal attack. The man who killed her, of course, was her husband.

WRONG ADDRESS

Sent to a call for a pregnant woman stabbed and in labor, the dispatcher gives the address of 235 2nd Avenue, third floor, apartment 3D. We arrive on scene to find that nobody there needed an ambulance. The dispatcher checks with the police on scene who confirm that there is a woman in labor and stabbed. They repeat their request to rush the bus. Again I inform the dispatcher there are no police on scene and no ambulance needed at our location. We check to ensure we are at the right address. The dispatcher repeats the address and sure enough, we are at the address given.

The dispatcher is upset with us for not finding the police or the patient. I again say there are no police or anyone needing an ambulance at the address.

We are still on the third floor when our back up calls up to me "George what do you need up stairs?" Being a bit upset with the dispatcher I tell him, "Joe, bring up a patient. We don't have one!"

We go down stairs to meet Joe and his partner. Joe is laughing about me telling him to bring up a patient.

Then the dispatcher advises us the address was in Brooklyn and the Brooklyn units were on scene.

BY NEW YORK CITY PARAMEDIC GEORGE STEFFENSEN

WRONG NUMBER

It was early in the morning when we were dispatched to 23rd Street and Broadway for the unconscious. This location is near a methadone clinic and we get a lot of people that have overdosed on their methadone.

As we pull up on scene, sure enough we see a male slumped over on the sidewalk. His name is Bill and we have picked him up so many times I can't even count.

I take one side and my partner takes the other as we basically drag him over to the ambulance where we can put him onto the bench seat. There, as always, we will give him a little Narcan, which will reverse the effects of the methadone and he will be back to normal.

A woman comes over to us as we are dragging Bill over to the bus and starts telling us to be careful with him, he may have had a stroke or maybe he is a diabetic.

One thing I don't need is a "concerned" bystander telling me how to do my job. The fact that she thinks this patient has had a stroke or diabetes is plain crazy talk. Obviously she doesn't know much about people on methadone. She also doesn't know Bill like we do. His only condition is his drug problem, which we know from taking him many times over the years.

Not being in a very good mood I tell her, "Thank you, we have it, you can go now!" That apparently wasn't what she wanted to hear so she comes closer. Again she tells me that she thinks he might be a diabetic and we should give him insulin. In a less-friendly voice I tell her, "Lady, you don't know what you're talking about. If you don't leave now I'm calling for an ambulance to take you in for psychiatric evaluation."

Things go downhill from here. "I want your supervisors number. I'm making a complaint!" she yells at me.

"You want me supervisors number?" I ask. "No problem. 1-800-SUCK MY DICK!" I close the door to the bus and go about working on poor Bill.

Later my boss will have me upstairs. He asks what happened on the call with Bill that someone had called to complain. I told him about the "lady" on scene causing problems, but Bill was still in the emergency room. He (as always) was very happy with our treatment.

He asked what number I gave her. I just smiled and said the usual number.

CANCER

So many times we are dispatched to different calls. Sometimes we get on scene, and the family members will tell us that the patient has cancer. This is, of course, important to know, but it doesn't tell us why the ambulance was called. Sometimes it's because the person has great pain or has trouble breathing; this would be the reason why the ambulance was called. The cancer might be the reason they have the pain or trouble breathing, but having cancer wasn't why they called.

I was working one day with my partner John. He is a great paramedic and a good friend. He moved away and he really is missed; he was one of the partners that made your day fun. I loved working with him but there were times that he made me a bit nervous with some of the crazy things he would do.

We are dispatched to a call for trouble breathing. We get to the scene and head up to the apartment. A family member answers the door and lets us into the apartment. John starts to ask some question to the patient as I prepare to take his vital signs.

John asks the patient, "Why did you call the ambulance?" The family member interrupts and tells John in a very soft voice, "He has cancer." John ignores the family member and repeats the question. "Sir, why did you call the ambulance?" Again the family member tells John in the soft voice, "He has cancer!"

And John says, in not a soft voice (as a matter of fact very loudly), "Well, he didn't get it this morning so why did you call an ambulance?"

The patient responded this time and let John know that he had trouble breathing. John continued and found out the patient was having chest pain. We place the patient on the monitor and see that he has significant elevations in several leads.

This patient's pain and trouble breathing has nothing to do with his cancer. He is having a heart attack. We work him up and quickly get him to the hospital.

He is lucky that he called when he did. He went up to the cath. lab where they opened up a clogged vessel, and he ends up doing fine.

John was famous for calling lymphoma "wimp-phoma." He would say, "Wimp-phoma? Hell, you can't even see that shit!"

THE BRAINS

One afternoon as I was working, I heard one of our new medics being sent to a job for an unconscious male. The police were asking for a rush; apparently the patient had been assaulted by a man with a bat. After hearing the police request for a rush, I listened to see what was going on, it sounded like a good job.

The new medic gives the 10-84 signal, which means they are on scene. Shortly after he has arrived on scene he requests backup. Requesting backup on a serious job is not unusual, however his request was not only unusual, but it was the funniest request that has ever come over the radio. In a frantic voice he screams over the radio, "Central, send me backup. His brains are coming out of his fucking head!"

After a moment of silence the dispatcher advised, "Backup is being sent but you can't say that over the air."

I looked over at my partner Jeff and ask him, "Jeff did you hear that request for back up?" Jeff was almost crying he was laughing so hard.

We all couldn't wait for the new medic to come back to the base so we could mess with him about his special backup request. Really, we just wanted to have some fun. This new medic was well liked and of course we all knew about getting excited on trauma jobs when we first start out.

BY NEW YORK CITY PARAMEDIC GEORGE STEFFENSEN

MURDER IN THE HALL

It is a hot summer night as my partner Hector and I stand outside our bus at St. Marks and 2nd Avenue. Although it is a Friday night, things are pretty slow. Then of course we get sent on a call, a stabbing at 874 10th Street, third floor hallway. We get into our bus and within a couple of minutes we are pulling up on scene.

I grab the oxygen, Hector grabs the stair chair and trauma bag and we head up to the third floor. This building is old and doesn't have an elevator. As we climb the stairs it is dark and dirty. I am ahead of Hector as we get to the third floor landing.

I see a big man laying on the floor in a big pool of blood. Quickly I check to see if he is breathing and has a pulse. He has neither! I call for a basic unit for backup for this traumatic arrest.

Hector and I start CPR on him. After the breathing tube is placed I do one man CPR as Hector cuts away his clothes so he can stop all this bleeding. The patient has deep stab wounds to his chest and back, which we cover with occlusive dressings. The basic unit arrives on scene; it is one of our units. We hear Alison ask over the radio, "What do you need upstairs?" Hector tells her, "Bring up a long board." We will carry him down on the board and be able to do CPR on the landings.

Then I notice something, I grab my portable radio: "Central, I need PD forthwith, 874 10th Street, third floor hallway!" Hector looks at me puzzled, not knowing why I'm putting over the emergency request for police.

I point to the blood trail on the floor. The blood trail starts from under the door at the apartment we are in front of. It is obvious that the stabbing victim had been in the apartment and had been dragged out into the hall. Looking at the size of the victim, who ever did this is someone I don't want to mess with.

Lucky for us, the police arrived in seconds. They were just outside the building as I was calling for them. Alison and Michelle bring up the long board. We quickly load the patient onto the long board and carry him down the stairs and into our bus.

Once the patient is in the ambulance, Alison and Michelle continue CPR while Hector gets the trauma lines ready. I get in front and am ready to drive to the trauma center. I warn my partners in the back that I'm ready to go. They yell up to me, "Go ahead!"

Within four minutes we are pulling into the trauma center. Michelle had called in the notification when we were bringing him down the stairs. Good thing she did it, as Hector and I both forgot to give it.

The trauma team works on the patient and they open his chest. He has large clumps of blood that fall out of his open chest. It looks like he was down for a while to have all that clotted blood in his chest cavity.

Shortly after opening his chest, the doctor in charge calls the code. Most traumatic arrests do not survive. He will not be one of the rare cases and is pronounced dead at 9:20 p.m.

Detectives from the 9th Precinct arrive as we are cleaning the back of our bloody ambulance. They need to get information from us for their report. They take our shield numbers and the ambulance call report number. We describe how the victim was positioned when we arrived. We also mentioned how the blood trail had lead into the apartment and that was when we called for emergency police response.

The detective said that we were right, the victim had been stabbed in that apartment by his brother. It was a sad story. The victim was a drug addict who kept coming to his brother's place. Stealing from his apartment when he wasn't home and now things were getting worse. The last two times before this happened, he came over and beat him and took any cash in the apartment. The poor guy just snapped and this time he wasn't going to be a victim any longer. When the brother pushed his way into the apartment he was ready with a big hunting knife. He stabbed and stabbed until he knew his brother could no longer torment him.

STABBINGS

THE BOWERY STABBING

My partner George and I were sent to 312 The Bowery (in front of that location) for the male stabbed. Something made us think that it could be a real job so we really did rush to the call. As I recall, this location is in a tough area, so a stabbing happening here won't surprise you. We arrived in a few minutes to find a man lying on the ground with blood coming from his chest. Wow, we were right; this was a real job. He has one stab wound to his left chest. We do a complete physical exam to ensure we don't miss any other injuries. We are treating the chest wound with an occlusive dressing, and his breathing is fine. George checks his lung sounds; they are clear and equal. As we are placing him onto the stretcher things turn very bad.

No not for the patient, but for me and my partner. From out of no-where, the man who had stabbed the patient is standing in front of us with a knife in his hand. He looked either crazy or on drugs, possibly both. He isn't a small man either. George quickly calls over his radio: "10-85 forthwith 312 Bowery, 10-85 forthwith 312 Bowery!" This means you need emergency help. You are in danger and you need police and any available units to respond to your location. What took only a minute or two will seem like a lifetime to me.

The man with the knife comes at me. He is too close for me to get away. I'm forced to fight for my life. He takes a swing at me with the knife. He just misses and I somehow grab his wrist. We struggle as I try desperately to get him to drop the knife. My partner is fighting too now as he joins in. I'm extremely lucky that George is a very strong guy. I couldn't have a better partner in this very bad situation. He is able to get the knife from him and throws it away. With the knife out of the equation we now have the advantage.

The guy reaches into his jacket and pulls out yet another knife. This one is longer and wider. He's still so close that turning to run is not an option

131

so I take a swing, punching him in the face. It is a good shot and I move in and grab his wrist again. From my training in the Marines I remembered this arm lock move and used this to keep him away from me. With the help of George we take him down to the ground. This hurts my shoulder and arm but I keep fighting. I end up on top of him. I have his arm and with all my strength I push his elbow back and it breaks. He drops the knife and my partner is holding him down with me.

The fight is over as units start screeching onto the scene; six ambulances and three police cars all ready to help. It's already done and we are basically all right. We continue back to our original patient. His chest wound is not to the pleural cavity and he is stable. We place a couple of IVs and give him oxygen. We monitor his vital signs and get him over to the trauma center.

One of the other units along with the police takes the bad guy to the hospital for his broken elbow. From there he will be charged with the assault and attempted murder of the guy he stabbed in the chest.

After we complete the call and my adrenalin has stopped pumping, I realize that my right shoulder hurts along with my right arm. During the struggle I was injured but was too scared to stop fighting or notice the pain. I tore my bicep muscle, ruptured my bicep tendon and had a massive rotator cuff tear. I will have to undergo four hours of surgery to put things back together. The good news is I still can work and play basketball. I know that it could have ended very differently and much worse. I still consider myself a lucky guy and still love the job.

Oh, and I have to laugh. This is pretty funny and I almost forgot it. Later, one of the guys who came to our aid, a little EMT who had rushed to help us, said (and let me remind you that I am 6'4", 230 lbs and my partner George is also a very big, strong guy, much stronger than I am) "You know as I was coming to help you I was thinking if you guys need help, what the hell am I going to do?" It made me laugh, but his coming even knowing that he would be putting himself in danger shows you that we have lots of heroic guys and gals here in EMS. This is another reason I love the job, because I know people will be there for me when I need help.

THE GIRL ON BROADWAY

Here we are, just finished some boring call. The night has been slow. Then a basic unit is dispatched to a stabbing on Broadway and 21st Street. I must have been on the job for a while, as I didn't try to "buff" the call.

The call is just a few blocks from where we were sitting. It did come over as a basic job so it could be just something minor like a cut arm. The basic unit arrives on scene very quickly as I hear them give the 88 signal. I do listen to them just in case it turns out to be something "real." The EMT requests medics for the patient. "Central, send us medics, we have an unconscious female in imminent arrest." Our unit responds and we are there in seconds. They are ventilating a young girl approximately 18-years-old who is unconscious and barely breathing. Her throat has been cut very deeply.

When her throat was slashed it severed her jugular vein and she had lost a lot of blood. The laceration is in fact so deep that when I position her to intubate her, I thought it might have cut into the trachea. She is in very critical condition. She has lost so much blood that we can't feel a radial pulse, which means her blood pressure is extremely low. She is on the verge of going into cardiac arrest. She needs to get to the trauma center now. Of course the airway has to be managed first. I carefully but quickly place the laryngoscope into her mouth so I can look into her throat to place the breathing tube. I also wanted to see if the trachea had been cut too. Thinking now the fact that I didn't see or hear air coming from the neck should have helped me realize her trachea was not cut. Besides, even if it is cut the tube should extend pass the cut and protect her airway.

With her airway taken care of we need to head over to the trauma center. En route to the hospital (which was only ten blocks away) my partner placed two large bore IVs while I was drove like a madman.

All this was done in under ten minutes from the time we got on scene to the time we were in the trauma slot. I was so amazed that my partner got both lines! Hell, I would have been impressed if my partner had gotten one line the way the bus was moving.

Anyway, the quick response of the basic unit, along with us being so close to the job worked in this young girl's favor. She will survive this terrible attack from an angry boyfriend.

THE BURNT MEDIC

The Burnt Medic. If you look it up in the dictionary, I'm sure you will find legendary Bruce Bell's picture there. Bruce is an original Harlem Paramedic with over 25 years on the streets.

I first met Bruce before I entered paramedic training. I was an emergency medical technician and was assigned to work with him up in Westchester. I laugh at the fact of how I was so impressed with him for being a city medic. He was very smart and very cocky. I loved it when he would tell the doctors to come help him lift the patients. Funnier still, as Bruce would direct things somehow when all was said and done Bruce was positioned in a way that he wasn't even near the patient when the lifting started. He always treated me well and of course when I became a medic and started working in the city I couldn't wait to throw his name around. 'I worked with Bruce Bell upstate," I would say. Unfortunately for me Bruce was already well known even back then as being too burnt.

However they would always say after the part that he was too burnt, before being on the streets too long Bruce Bell was one of the top paramedics anywhere.

I remember doing a transport call with Bruce for the private service, a pediatric transport with the pediatric team from a big hospital. They always had the EMT and medic carry everything as they walked empty handed behind us.

On this day Bruce gave me a bag and he took a smaller bag. He looked at the doctor and told him to bring the rest of the stuff if he wants to bring it. I was a bit in shock but Bruce pointed out that, "It says Paramedic, not pack mule on the back of my jacket!"

Other things I have heard while working opposite Bruce; on a different city unit, the dispatcher called saying Bruce's unit was too long on scene. The dispatcher said, "X-ray unit, I show you on scene 47 minutes!" Bruce replies, "Central, that's no record for me."

Another time Bruce gave a notification that his patient was in shock but had no IV access. Some new medic asked over the air if he needed medic back up. Bruce calmly replied, "When I was a rookie that might have meant something."

Like I said, Bruce has been working as a medic for over 25 years, but what is even crazier is he has been working two jobs and more for that whole time. So I say he deserves to take it a bit easy. You have to respect him. I certainly do.

I'm not sure if I want him working on me. Hell, with him responding I could die of old age before he gets to me.

All kidding aside, I do respect him and am proud to know him.

15 YEARS ON THE STREETS

So here I am today, over 15 years on the streets working as a paramedic. I have surely seen more then my share of things people shouldn't see. I look in the mirror to see the physical changes that have come.

I started working as a medic when I was thirty-three. I'm now over fifty with gray hair. My body has been to hell and back. I injured my knee on a call and needed surgery to repair that. I have scars on both legs where I had vascular surgery. I have a big scar around my right shoulder; I needed that after I was assaulted at the stabbing on the Bowery. My right bicep muscle was torn and is deformed as well, it was torn during the assault too. The eagerness on my face when the dispatcher calls my unit is no longer there. More an expression of what now? shows on my tired face.

The mental changes are there as well. Funny, when I first started out I never thought that I would be bored with the trauma jobs, and now I look at it as too much work. Thinking what a pain in the ass cleaning up afterward is going to be. A far cry from when I took pride and thought it was so cool to have the back of my bus look like a slaughterhouse. Going on calls now, I just hope it will be something simple. Something that I won't need to do much.

Carrying all this equipment up flights of stairs is much harder today then when I started out. The first thing is that I don't want to use the equipment any longer. Secondly, most of the time I won't need to use it, which I had not realized when I was rookie buff. Plus, carrying all this heavy equipment hurts my knees going up stairs. Hell, they hurt going up stairs without all this junk. When I was more caring, the adrenalin rush could get me past the pain, but now I no longer get that rush and the pain is very real. I notice every step as we go up all these stairs. Knowing full well that once we reach the patient it will be for some nonsense.

I no longer care about the saves as I once did. Yes, it is still good to save someone, but back then it was about me too. Look I saved someone, aren't I a great medic!

Is it that I have been on the streets too long or has my age finally made me realize that the calls are just about the patients? No one cares about the paramedics.

When I started out being the guy who saved the patient, being the "hero" is what I really wanted to be. Now I want to be the guy on the cancellation. I want to be on the simple call where I don't need to do much, if anything at all.

I enjoy helping others even today. So I guess what I am saying is that the coolness of the job has worn off. The glory days have come and gone. Let the new guys save the day. I see the new medics with their buff belts ready to save the world, as I was when I started out. They are here and they will do a great job. I will try to remember what it was to be the rookie medic. I will try my best to take these rookies under my wing, as the good medics did for me.

No more buff belt for me. No Mag-Lite hanging there. No window punch ready to gain access into a car. No more pouch for my gloves. No equipment of any kind hanging on me now. It is all with the rest of the equipment in the ambulance where it belongs. It is close enough to do a good job.

I'm not a bad guy. I'm just not as excited about the job as I once was. The years of doing ninety percent nonsense will take a toll on anyone.

Hard to believe, but even today I really do think being a paramedic was a good choice for me. That small ten percent of the "real jobs" where I made a difference makes me feel good. It is really a great feeling when you know that your actions played a part in someone having more time with their families.

THE FINAL CHAPTER

I have had a great time working as a paramedic. I'm not retired yet, so maybe I can write more stories another time. Reflecting back to the early days and recounting the different jobs I've done over the years has been fun for me and my family. This book writing gave me a chance to share what my job has been about. Through the changes in me, and maybe by hearing some of the stories, people can see a little what being a medic is all about.

Of course, reading or hearing the stories can't get you to see it completely. My brother gave me a great example when I asked him what Marine boot camp was going to be like. He told me, "I can tell you it burns to put your hand into a fire, but until your hand is in the fire you can't really understand what it is like." He was right. As I was getting off the bus at Paris Island with the drill instructors screaming Get off the bus! Get off the bus! at 4:00 a.m., I understood the feeling of the fire.

I really want to thank everyone who has been there for me, all the people that I've been with from my early training days, through the changes, to my semi-burnt days now. Just thinking of all the different calls; the good ones and even the bad ones were all something I will never forget. From being so nervous as a new medic to being the hero, to now just being a simple medic trying to keep doing the right thing.

I know I've said this a lot but I am truly a very lucky man. Working at a job that I love, and having so much support from family, friends, partners and even co-workers.

I hope to be remembered as a good husband, a good father, and good grandfather. And after that, not to be remembered as some great paramedic, but as a good partner and friend.

Made in the USA
Lexington, KY
06 August 2016